HANDBOOK OF COMMON ORTHOPAEDIC FRACTURES

Second Edition

Scott Hal Kozin, M.D.
Department of Orthopaedics
Mayo Clinic and Mayo Foundation
Rochester, Minnesota

Anthony Clayton Berlet, M.D.
Department of Plastic and Reconstructive Surgery
UMDNJ - New Jersey Medical School
Newark, New Jersey

1992

HANDBOOK OF COMMON ORTHOPAEDIC FRACTURES

Second Edition

Copyright © 1992, 1989 by Medical Surveillance Inc., P.O. Box 1629, West Chester, PA. All Rights Reserved. Printed in the United States of America.

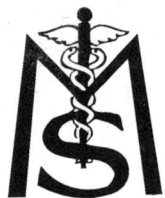

The Authors or Publisher are not responsible for typographical errors within the contents of this booklet.

Illustrations by Anthony C. Berlet, M.D.

TABLE OF CONTENTS

PAGE

INTRODUCTION 1

UPPER EXTREMITY 3
   DISTAL PHALANX FRACTURES 4
   BASE OF THUMB METACARPAL FRACTURES 6
   SCAPHOID FRACTURES 12
   FRACTURES OF THE DISTAL RADIUS 14
   FRACTURES OF THE PROXIMAL ULNA WITH RADIAL HEAD
      DISLOCATION - MONTEGGIA LESION 20
   FRACTURES OF THE OLECRANON 22
   CORONOID FRACTURES 24
   FRACTURES OF THE RADIAL HEAD 26
   FRACTURES OF THE DISTAL HUMERUS 28
   FRACTURES OF THE HUMERAL CONDYLES 30
   CAPITELLUM FRACTURES 32
   INTERCONDYLAR FRACTURES OF THE HUMERUS 34
   TRANSCONDYLAR FRACTURES OF THE HUMERUS 36
   SUPRACONDYLAR FRACTURES OF THE HUMERUS 38
   FRACTURES OF THE PROXIMAL HUMERUS 40
   FRACTURES OF THE CLAVICLE 48
   FRACTURES OF THE SCAPULA 52

SPINE 59
   CLASSIFICATION OF CERVICAL SPINE INJURIES 60
   FRACTURES OF THE ODONTOID PROCESS 72
   THORACOLUMBAR SPINAL INJURY CLASSIFICATION 74

PAGE

PELVIS AND ACETABULUM 83
- CLASSIFICATION OF PELVIC DISRUPTION 84
- CLASSIFICATION OF ACETABULUM FRACTURES 94
- SACRAL FRACTURE CLASSIFICATION 102

LOWER EXTREMITY 105
- CLASSIFICATION OF HIP FRACTURES 106
- FRACTURES OF THE FEMORAL NECK 108
- INTERTROCHANTERIC HIP FRACTURES 110
- SUBTROCHANTERIC FRACTURES OF THE FEMUR 112
- FEMORAL SHAFT FRACTURES 118
- SUPRACONDYLAR FEMORAL FRACTURES 120
- PATELLA FRACTURES 128
- FRACTURES OF THE TIBIAL SPINE 130
- FRACTURES OF THE TIBIAL PLATEAU 132
- TIBIAL SHAFT FRACTURES 138
- FRACTURES OF THE DISTAL TIBIA WITH INTRA-ARTICULAR EXTENSION - PILON FRACTURE 140
- ANKLE FRACTURE CLASSIFICATIONS 142
- FRACTURES OF THE NECK OF THE TALUS 152
- TALAR BODY FRACTURES 154
- FRACTURES OF THE CALCANEUS 156
- CLASSIFICATION OF OPEN FRACTURES 162

EPONYMS 165

REFERENCES 213
INDEX 221
ORDER FORM 225

PREFACE

Orthopaedic surgery is a field of medicine that encompasses a wide spectrum of disease entities and fractures. Fractures may occur anywhere in the human body, and accurate assessment is essential for diagnosis and treatment. Fractures throughout the body have been extensively analyzed and classified. These classifications are based on fracture configurations, mechanism of injury, or fracture stability. This has led to an overwhelming number of classifications and eponyms which are frequently confusing and cumbersome. In addition, many fractures have multiple classifications creating further confusion. A classification should provide therapeutic and prognostic information to be valuable in fracture management.

The second edition of the **HANDBOOK OF COMMON ORTHOPAEDIC FRACTURES** is published for the practicing physician, resident, medical student and other health professionals to simplify fracture classifications, help access fracture stability, and direct treatment. All fractures should initially be described according to length, angulation, rotation, displacement, and degree of comminution, prior to attempting specific classification. These variables are essential in orthopaedic analysis for treatment of fractures and are incorporated in many of the classification schemas. This handbook contains the majority of fractures that have been appropriately classified and includes an eponym section for reference purposes. Extremely uncommon fractures and those without adequate classification are not included in this text.

This handbook is organized into five sections: (1) Upper Extremity, (2) Spine, (3) Pelvis and Acetabulum, (4) Lower Extremity, and (5) Eponyms. The fracture classifications are listed in a distal to proximal direction for the Upper Extremity followed by a cephalad to caudad direction for the remaining sections. The Eponym section is listed in alphabetical order. This organization is designed to allow quick and easy reference to specific fracture classifications.

The **HANDBOOK OF COMMON ORTHOPAEDIC FRACTURES, Second Edition**, is physically designed to fit in a pocket to allow for easy accessibility. We hope this text will be useful in simplifying fracture assessment and classifications. We welcome any suggestions, comments, and criticisms that may improve our handbook.

We wish to thank Edward J. Barbieri, Ph.D., and G. John DiGregorio, M.D., Ph.D., for their assistance with the composition and preparation of this handbook.

Scott H. Kozin, M.D.
Anthony C. Berlet, M.D.

INTRODUCTION

Orthopaedic fracture management begins with initial patient evaluation. The entire patient and involved extremity should be carefully and thoroughly examined. A complete neurovascular examination of the potentially fractured extremity is vital in the initial assessment. Neurovascular compromise is an orthopaedic emergency and requires prompt therapeutic intervention. All fractures should be initially splinted to prevent further tissue damage and for patient comfort. The skin should be inspected for evidence of bone penetration leading to open fracture management. Open fractures require cultures, debridement, antibiotics, and sterile dressings as part of their initial management. Radiographic analysis should be prompt and should include the joint above and below the fracture; for example, a femoral shaft fracture should have radiographic visualization of the entire femur including the femoral head and condyles.

After careful history, physical examination, and radiography, an appropriate description of the fracture should be formulated. Orthopaedic fracture description is based upon length, angulation, rotation, and degree of bony comminution. A fractured extremity may be shortened or distracted, angulated in multiple directions, malrotated, or severely comminuted. All of these factors influence the therapeutic decision process and effect overall prognosis. Fractures should also be described as open with bone penetration of the skin or closed with preservation of the overlying skin. Fracture description should include the overlying soft tissue damage as well as the disruption of underlying bone and neurovascular elements. These variables all are indicative of the amount of energy absorbed by the fractured extremity at the time of injury. These factors are major determinants in the overall prognosis of the injured extremity.

Many fractures have been organized into classification schemas to provide therapeutic and prognostic information valuable in fracture management. This second edition text organizes those orthopaedic classifications into four expanded sections:

(1) Upper Extremity,
(2) Spine,
(3) Pelvis and Acetabulum, and
(4) Lower Extremity.

The Upper Extremity classifications are listed in a distal to proximal direction beginning with distal phalangeal fractures and progressing proximally including Frykman's classification of wrist fractures, Mason's classifications of radial head fractures, and Neer's classification of proximal humeral fractures. Each fracture classification is accompanied by extensive illustrations to aid in the understanding and application of specific classification schemas.

The Spine section progresses from a cephalad to caudad direction and includes cervical and thoracolumbar fractures. There is a separate section dedicated to odontoid fractures with illustrations in both the anteroposterior and lateral views.

The third section concentrates on pelvis and acetabular fractures. Tile's classification of pelvic disruption and acetabular fractures was selected because of its valuable therapeutic and prognostic information. This classification is presented in outline form with detailed illustrations to simplify its application in the clinical setting.

The fourth section involves the entire lower extremity beginning with hip fractures. These fractures are divided into femoral neck, intertrochanteric and subtrochanteric classifications. Accurate classification of these common fractures is necessary to select appropriate treatment. This section lists fractures in a superior to inferior direction and includes Winquist's classification of femoral shaft comminution, Hawkin's classification of talar neck fractures, and Essex-Lopresti's classification of calcaneus fractures. Ankle fractures are commonly classified according to either the Lauge-Hansen or AO schema. Therefore, both of these classifications are included in this text.

The fifth section of this handbook is dedicated to fracture eponyms. Eponyms to describe various fracture configurations are commonly employed. An alphabetical listing of fracture eponyms with illustrations and references is presented to allow easy accessibility.

The organization into these various sections is to allow an easily accessible reference text to specific fracture classifications and eponyms. The detailed illustrations are to simplify the understanding of these classification schemas. Hopefully, this combination of text and illustrations will simplify orthopaedic fracture classifications and be useful in the clinical setting.

UPPER EXTREMITY

DISTAL PHALANX FRACTURES

(Kaplan Classification)

I. LONGITUDINAL

II. TRANSVERSE

III. COMMINUTED

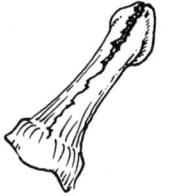

I. Longitudinal

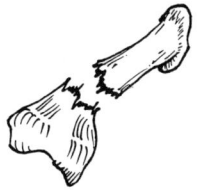

II. Transverse

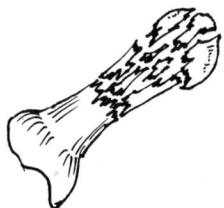

III. Comminuted

BASE OF THUMB METACARPAL FRACTURES

(Green Classification)

INTRA-ARTICULAR FRACTURES

    I.   BENNETT'S FRACTURE

    II.   ROLANDO'S FRACTURE

EXTRA-ARTICULAR FRACTURES

    III.   FRACTURES OF THE METACARPAL BASE

        A.   TRANSVERSE

        B.   OBLIQUE

    IV.   EPIPHYSEAL FRACTURE

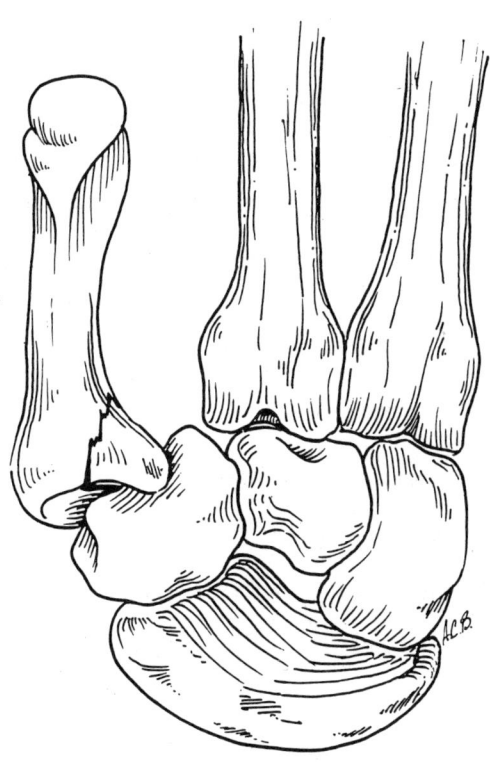

BASE OF THUMB METACARPAL FRACTURES

(Green Classification)

INTRA-ARTICULAR FRACTURES

    I.   BENNETT'S FRACTURE

    II.   ROLANDO'S FRACTURE

BENNETT'S and ROLANDO's FRACTURES are further described in the EPONYM SECTION.

I. Bennett's Fracture

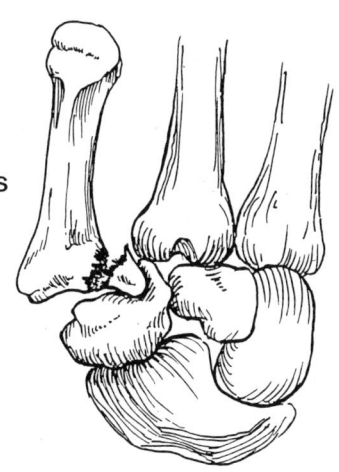

II. Rolando's Fracture

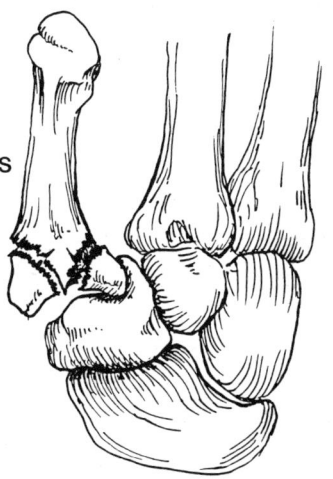

BASE OF THUMB METACARPAL FRACTURES

(Green Classification)

EXTRA-ARTICULAR FRACTURES

    III.   FRACTURES OF THE METACARPAL BASE

           A.   TRANSVERSE

           B.   OBLIQUE

    IV.   EPIPHYSEAL FRACTURE

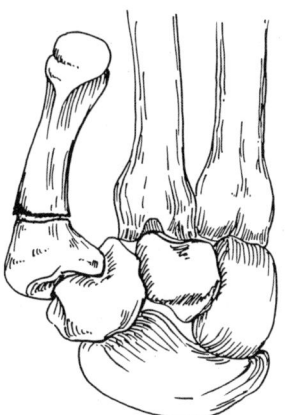

IIIA. Transverse

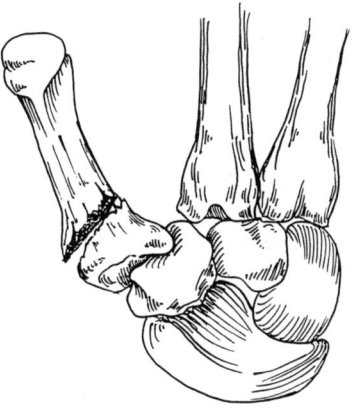

IIIB. Oblique

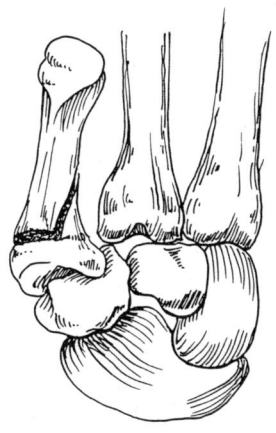

IV. Epiphyseal

SCAPHOID FRACTURES

(Russe Classification)

ANATOMIC LOCATION

    I.   PROXIMAL THIRD - 20%[a]

    II.   MIDDLE THIRD - 70%

    III.   DISTAL THIRD - 10%

FRACTURE CONFIGURATION

    I.   TRANSVERSE

    II.   VERTICAL OBLIQUE

    III.   HORIZONTAL OBLIQUE

Proximal third scaphoid fractures have increased incidence of avascular necrosis.

Forces across the wrist tend to compress and stabilize the horizontal oblique and transverse scaphoid fractures. The vertical oblique configuration tends to displace as the forces shear the fracture surface.

[a] *Percentages indicate the frequency of fracture occurrence.*

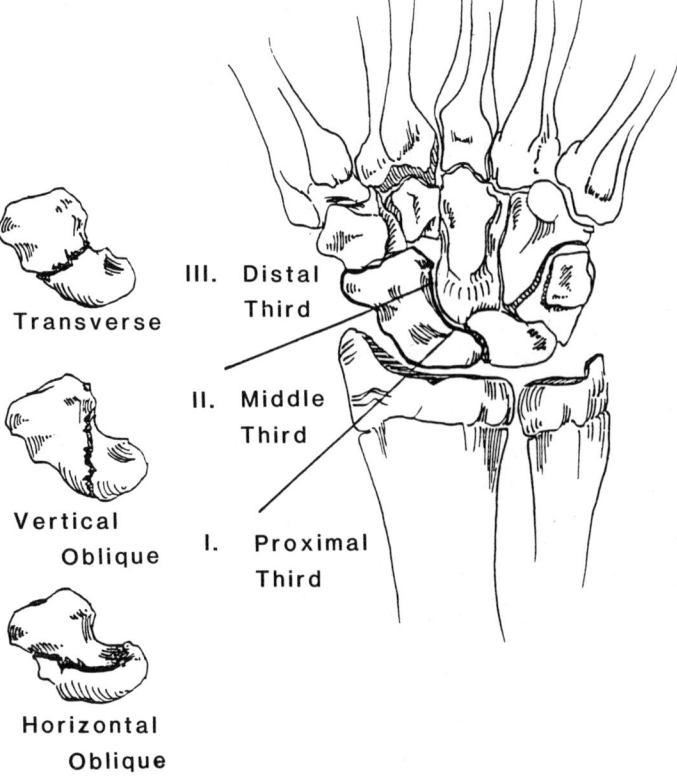

Transverse

Vertical Oblique

Horizontal Oblique

III. Distal Third

II. Middle Third

I. Proximal Third

FRACTURES OF THE DISTAL RADIUS

(Frykman Classification)

FRACTURE PATTERN	DISTAL ULNA FRACTURE	
	ABSENT	PRESENT
EXTRA-ARTICULAR	I	II
INTRA-ARTICULAR INVOLVING RADIOCARPAL JOINT	III	IV
INTRA-ARTICULAR INVOLVING RADIOULNAR JOINT	V	VI
INTRA-ARTICULAR INVOLVING RADIOCARPAL and RADIOULNAR JOINTS	VII	VIII

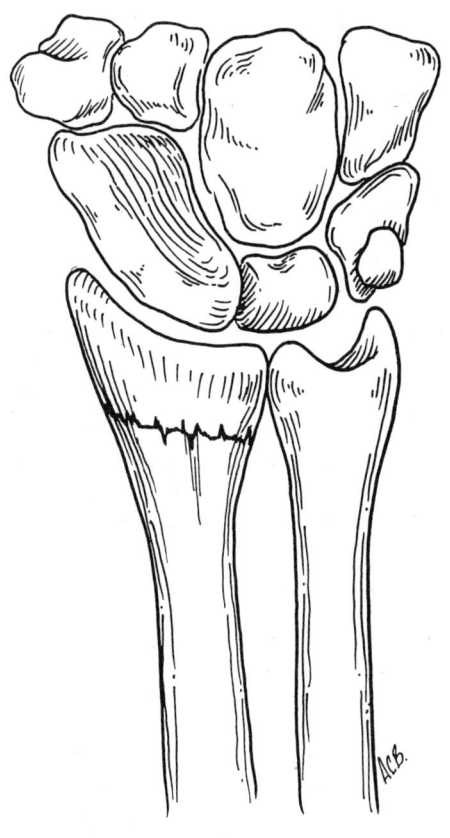

FRACTURES OF THE DISTAL RADIUS

(Frykman Classification)

FRACTURE PATTERN	DISTAL ULNA FRACTURE	
	ABSENT	PRESENT
EXTRA-ARTICULAR	I	II
INTRA-ARTICULAR INVOLVING RADIOCARPAL JOINT	III	IV

I.

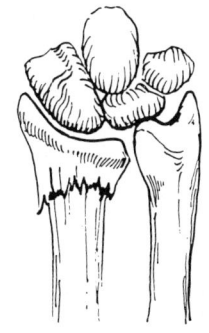

II.

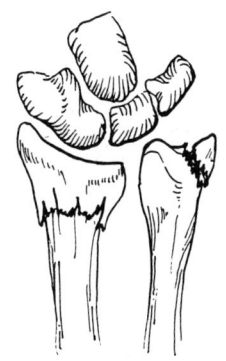

III.

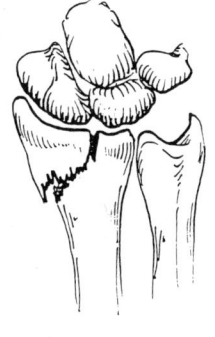

IV.

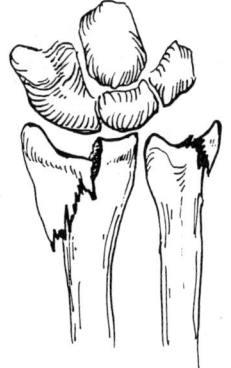

FRACTURES OF THE DISTAL RADIUS

(Frykman Classification)

FRACTURE PATTERN	DISTAL ULNA FRACTURE	
	ABSENT	PRESENT
INTRA-ARTICULAR INVOLVING RADIOULNAR JOINT	V	VI
INTRA-ARTICULAR INVOLVING RADIOCARPAL and RADIOULNAR JOINTS	VII	VIII

V.

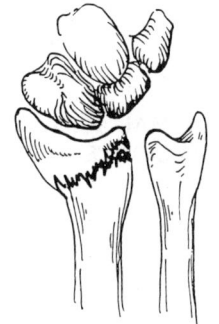

VI.

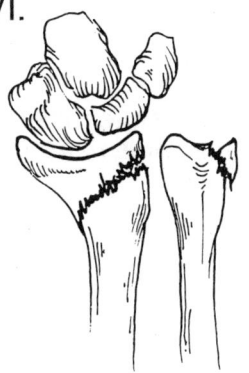

VII.

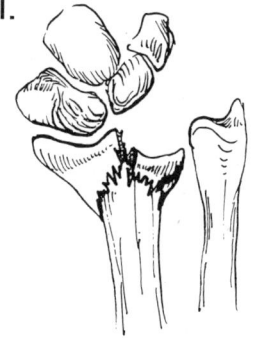

VIII.

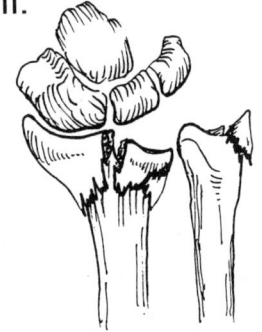

FRACTURES OF THE PROXIMAL ULNA
WITH RADIAL HEAD DISLOCATION - MONTEGGIA LESION

(Bado Classification)

I. ANTERIOR DISLOCATION OF THE RADIAL HEAD AND FRACTURE OF THE ULNAR DIAPHYSIS AT ANY LEVEL WITH ANTERIOR ANGULATION

II. POSTERIOR OR POSTEROLATERAL DISLOCATION OF THE RADIAL HEAD AND FRACTURE OF THE ULNAR DIAPHYSIS WITH POSTERIOR ANGULATION

III. LATERAL OR ANTEROLATERAL DISLOCATION OF THE RADIAL HEAD AND FRACTURE OF THE ULNAR METAPHYSIS

IV. ANTERIOR DISLOCATION OF THE RADIAL HEAD, FRACTURE OF THE THE PROXIMAL THIRD OF THE RADIUS, AND FRACTURE OF THE THE ULNA AT THE SAME LEVEL

Type I fracture dislocation is the most common type, accounting for approximately 65 percent of Monteggia lesions. Type IV lesions are uncommon, less than 5 percent of total.

I.

II.

III.

IV.

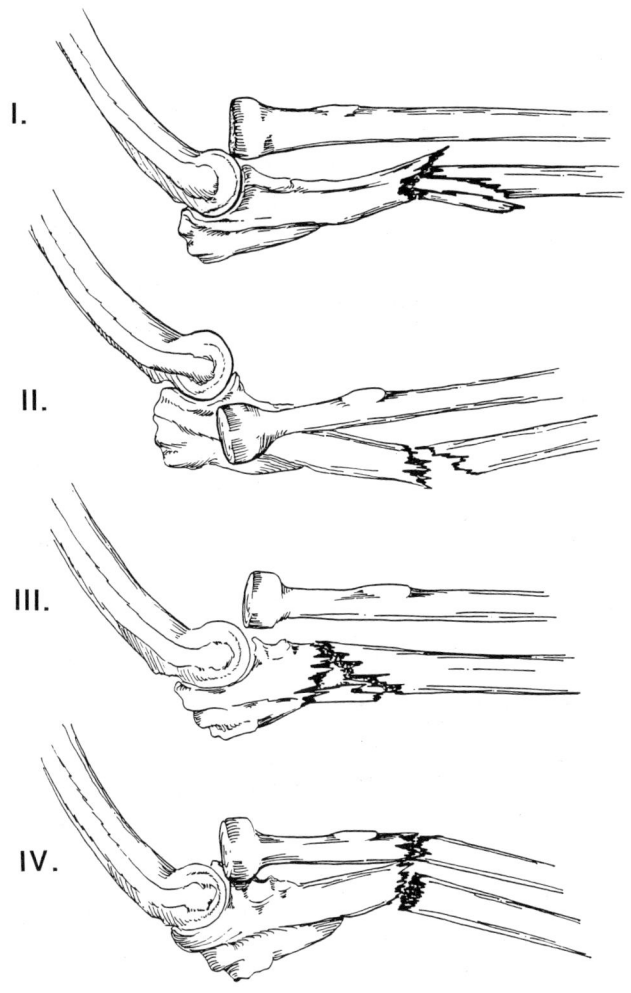

21

FRACTURES OF THE OLECRANON

(Colton Classification)

I. UNDISPLACED FRACTURES

II. DISPLACED FRACTURES

    A. AVULSION FRACTURES

    B. OBLIQUE AND TRANSVERSE FRACTURES

    C. COMMINUTED FRACTURES

    D. FRACTURE DISLOCATIONS

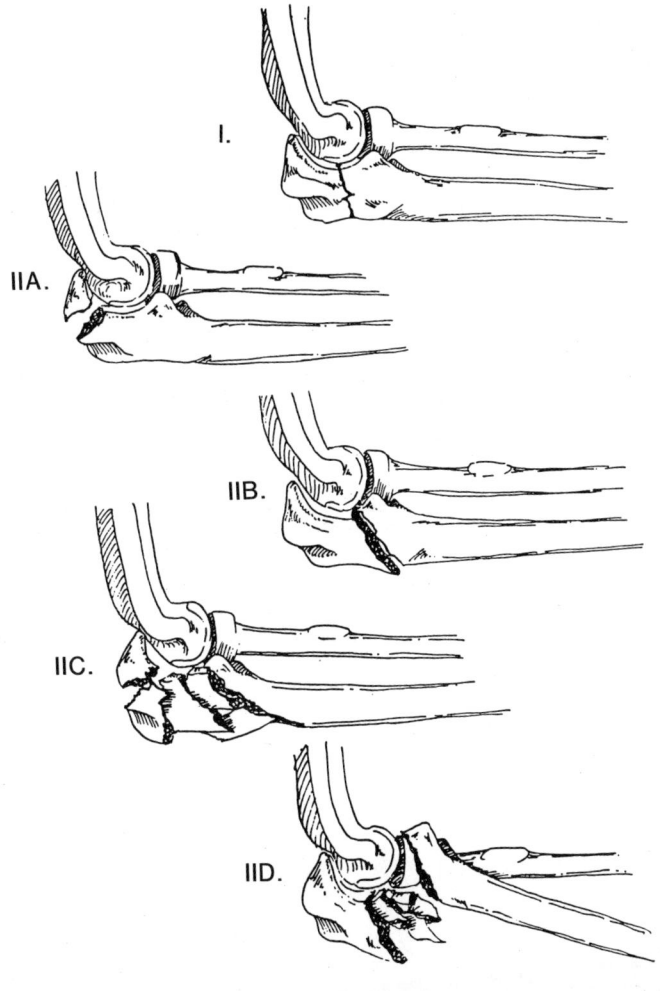

CORONOID FRACTURES

(Morrey Classification)

I. AVULSION OF THE TIP OF THE CORONOID PROCESS

II. SINGLE OR COMMINUTED FRAGMENT INVOLVING 50 PERCENT OR LESS OF THE CORONOID PROCESS

III. SINGLE OR COMMINUTED FRAGMENT INVOLVING GREATER THAN 50 PERCENT OF THE CORONOID PROCESS

Coronoid fractures are uncommon and often associated with elbow dislocations.

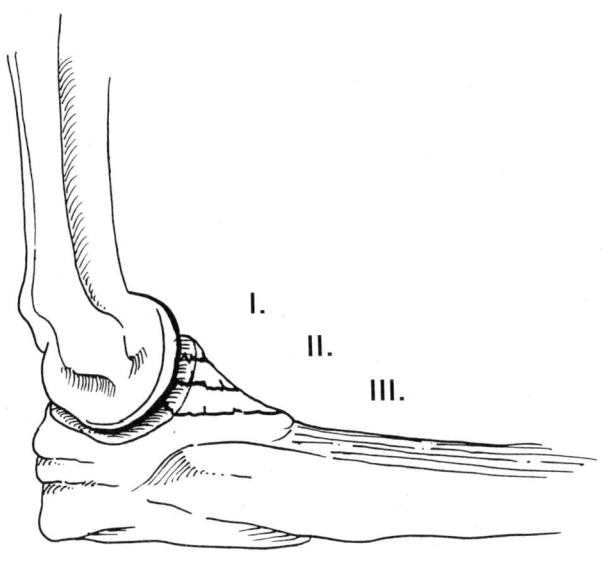

FRACTURES OF THE RADIAL HEAD

(Mason Classification with Johnston Modification)

I. NONDISPLACED LINEAR OR TRANSVERSE FRACTURES - 50%[a]

II. FRACTURES WITH MINIMAL DISPLACEMENT OR COMMINUTED FRACTURES WITHOUT DISPLACEMENT - 20%

III. COMMINUTED FRACTURES WITH MARKED DISPLACEMENT - 20%

IV. RADIAL HEAD FRACTURES WITH ELBOW DISLOCATION - 10%

Most common elbow fracture in adults.

[a] *Percentages indicate the frequency of fracture occurrence.*

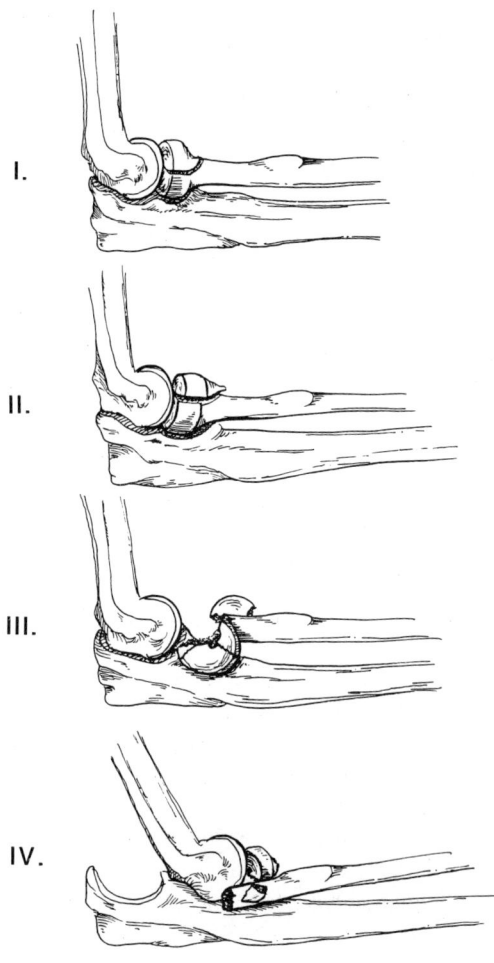

FRACTURES OF THE DISTAL HUMERUS

(Muller Classification)

A. EXTRA-ARTICULAR FRACTURES

    A1. AVULSION FRACTURES OF THE EPICONDYLES

    A2. SIMPLE SUPRACONDYLAR FRACTURE

    A3. COMMINUTED SUPRACONDYLAR FRACTURE

B. INTRA-ARTICULAR FRACTURES OF ONE CONDYLE

    B1. FRACTURE OF THE TROCHLEA

    B2. FRACTURE OF THE CAPITELLUM

    B3. TANGENTIAL FRACTURE OF THE TROCHLEA

C. BI-CONDYLAR FRACTURES

    C1. Y-FRACTURE

    C2. Y-FRACTURE WITH SUPRACONDYLAR COMMINUTION

    C3. COMMINUTED FRACTURE

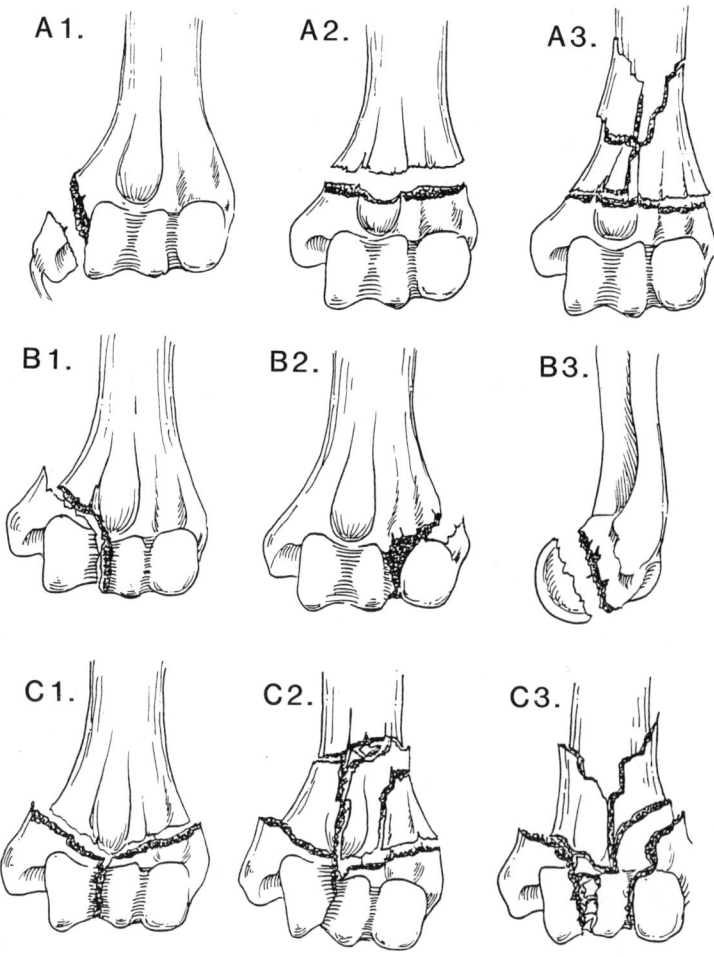

FRACTURES OF THE HUMERAL CONDYLES

(Milch Classification)

LATERAL HUMERAL CONDYLE

I. SIMPLE FRACTURE OF THE LATERAL CONDYLE WITH LATERAL WALL OF TROCHLEA ATTACHED TO MAIN MASS OF THE HUMERUS

II. FRACTURE WITH LATERAL WALL OF TROCHLEA ATTACHED TO FRACTURED LATERAL CONDYLAR FRAGMENT

MEDIAL LATERAL CONDYLE

I. SIMPLE FRACTURE OF MEDIAL CONDYLE WITH LATERAL WALL OF TROCHLEA ATTACHED TO MAIN MASS OF THE HUMERUS

II. FRACTURE WITH LATERAL WALL OF TROCHLEA ATTACHED TO FRACTURED MEDIAL CONDYLAR FRAGMENT

Type II fractures involve the trochlea and are unstable.

Lateral Medial

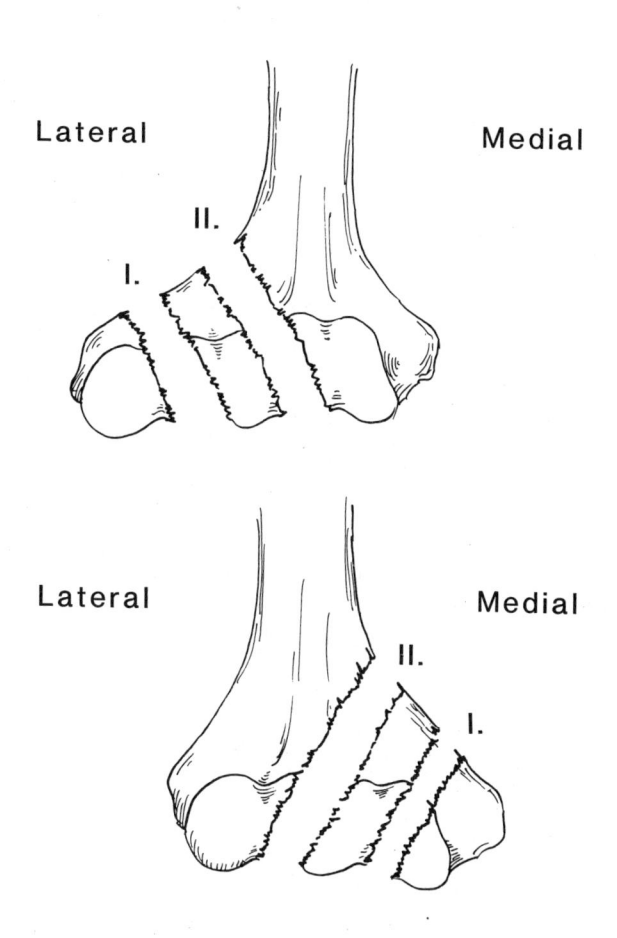

I. II.

Lateral Medial

II. I.

31

CAPITELLUM FRACTURES

(Bryan and Morrey Classification)

I. CAPITELLUM FRACTURE THAT INVOLVES THE MAJORITY OF THE OSSEOUS PORTION AND MAY EXTEND INTO ADJACENT TROCHLEA

II. SLICE FRACTURE OF THE CAPITELLUM WITH VARIABLE AMOUNT OF ARTICULAR CARTILAGE AND MINIMAL SUBCHONDRAL BONE

III. COMMINUTED OR COMPRESSION FRACTURE

Type I is the most common capitellum fracture.

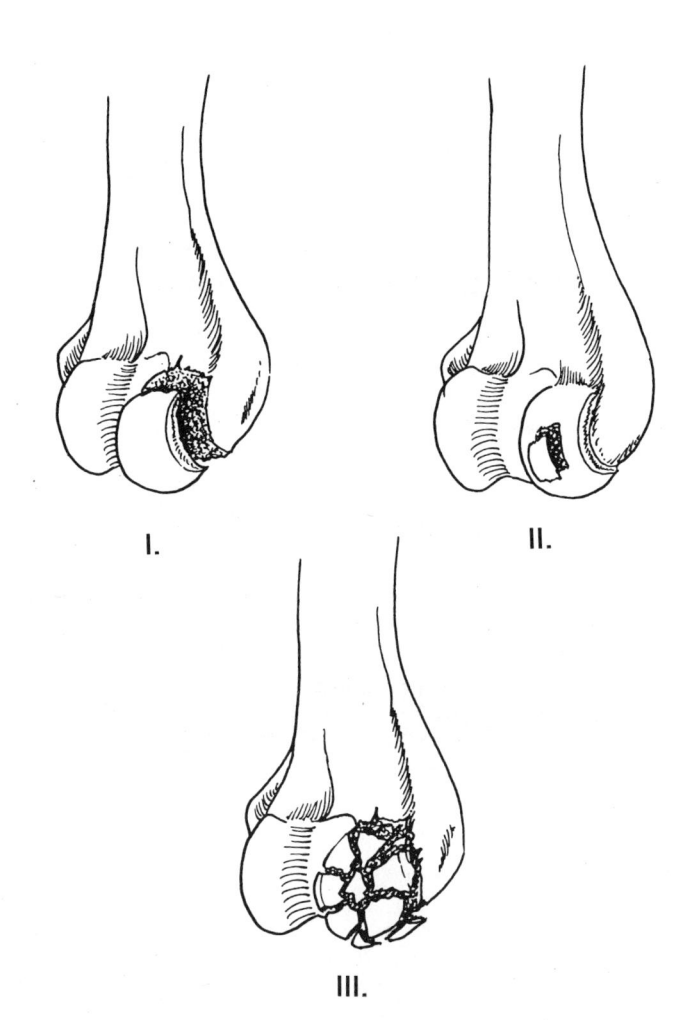

I.

II.

III.

INTERCONDYLAR FRACTURES OF THE HUMERUS

(Riseborough and Radin Classification)

I. NO DISPLACEMENT OF THE FRAGMENTS

II. T-SHAPED FRACTURE WITH THE TROCHLEAR AND CAPITELLAR FRAGMENTS SEPARATED BUT NOT APPRECIABLY ROTATED IN THE FRONTAL PLANE

III. T-SHAPED FRACTURE WITH SEPARATION OF THE FRAGMENTS AND SIGNIFICANT ROTARY DEFORMITY

IV. T-SHAPED INTERCONDYLAR FRACTURES WITH SEVERE COMMINUTION OF THE ARTICULAR SURFACE AND WIDE SEPARATION OF THE HUMERUS CONDYLES

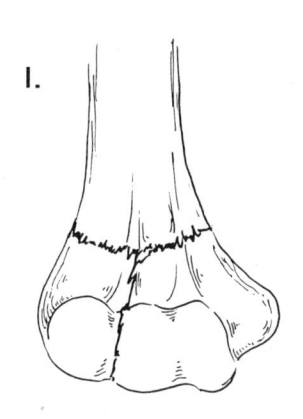

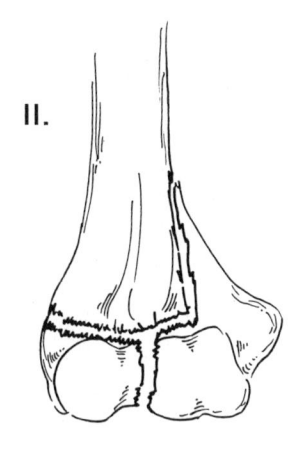

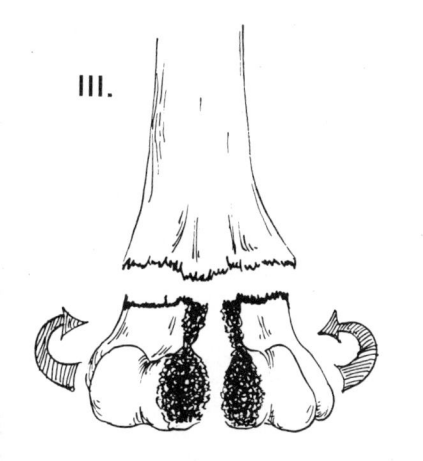

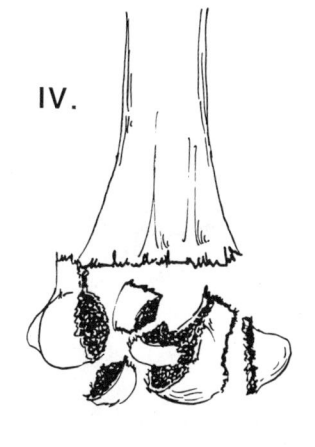

I.

II.

III.

IV.

TRANSCONDYLAR FRACTURES OF THE HUMERUS

(Ashurst Classification)

I. POSTERIOR DISPLACEMENT

II. ANTERIOR DISPLACEMENT

TRANSCONDYLAR FRACTURES are intercapsular fractures through the condyles. Displacement of the dicondylar fragment is usually posterior.

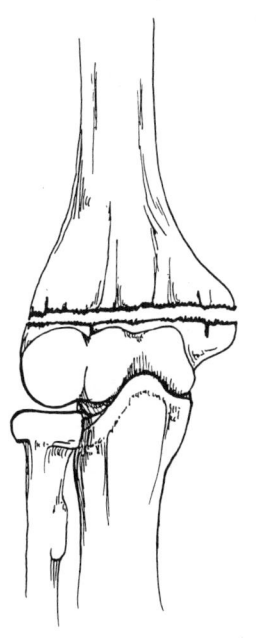

Transcondylar

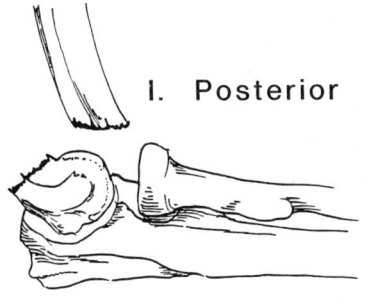

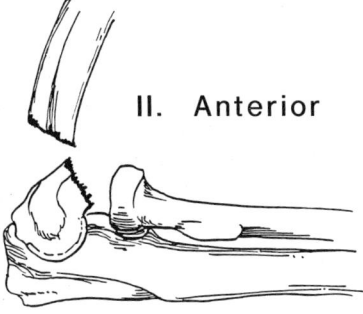

I. Posterior

II. Anterior

SUPRACONDYLAR FRACTURES OF THE HUMERUS

(Modified Kocher Classification)

I. EXTENSION TYPE

II. FLEXION TYPE

SUPRACONDYLAR EXTENSION FRACTURES are more common than the FLEXION TYPE and approximately 50 percent are completely displaced.

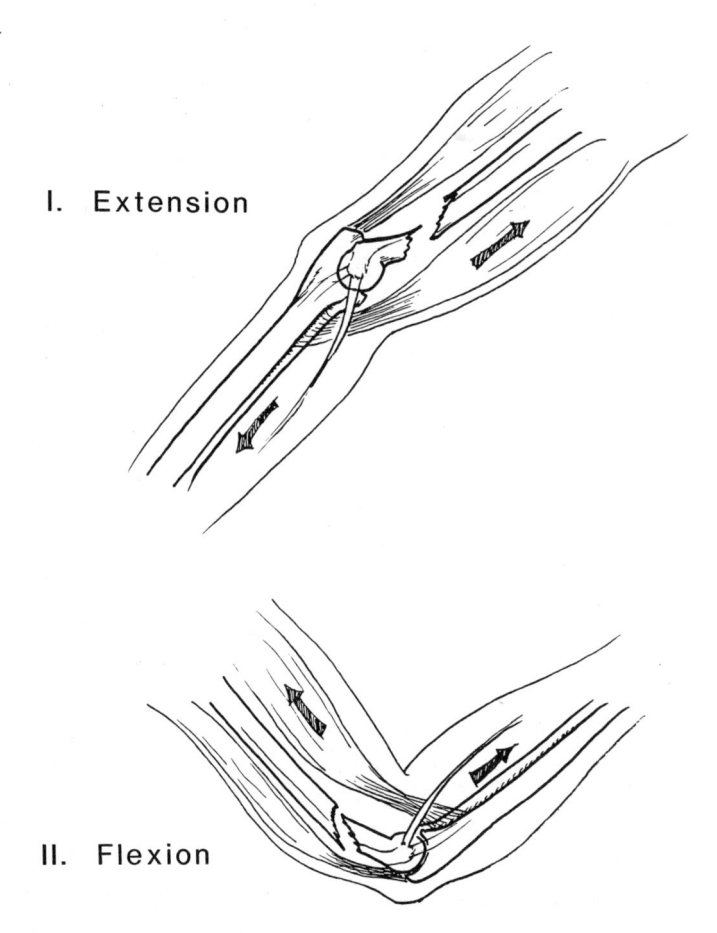

I. Extension

II. Flexion

FRACTURES OF THE PROXIMAL HUMERUS

(Neer Classification)

I. ONE-PART OR MINIMALLY DISPLACED FRACTURE WHERE NO SEGMENTS ARE DISPLACED BY 1.0 CM OR ANGULATED BY 45 DEGREES

II. TWO-PART FRACTURE WHERE ONE SEGMENT IS SIGNIFICANTLY DISPLACED BY 1.0 CM OR 45 DEGREES

III. THREE-PART FRACTURE WHERE TWO SEGMENTS ARE SIGNIFICANTLY DISPLACED BY 1.0 CM OR 45 DEGREES

IV. FOUR-PART FRACTURE WHERE ALL FOUR MAJOR SEGMENTS ARE DISPLACED BY 1.0 CM OR 45 DEGREES

V. FRACTURE DISLOCATION

Classification based on four fracture segments: (1) the articular segment, (2) the greater tuberosity, (3) the lesser tuberosity, and (4) the humeral shaft.

Classification describes only displaced segments which are defined as 1.0 cm displacement or 45 degree angulation.

Multiple fracture configurations are possible.

80 percent of PROXIMAL HUMERAL FRACTURES are minimally displaced.

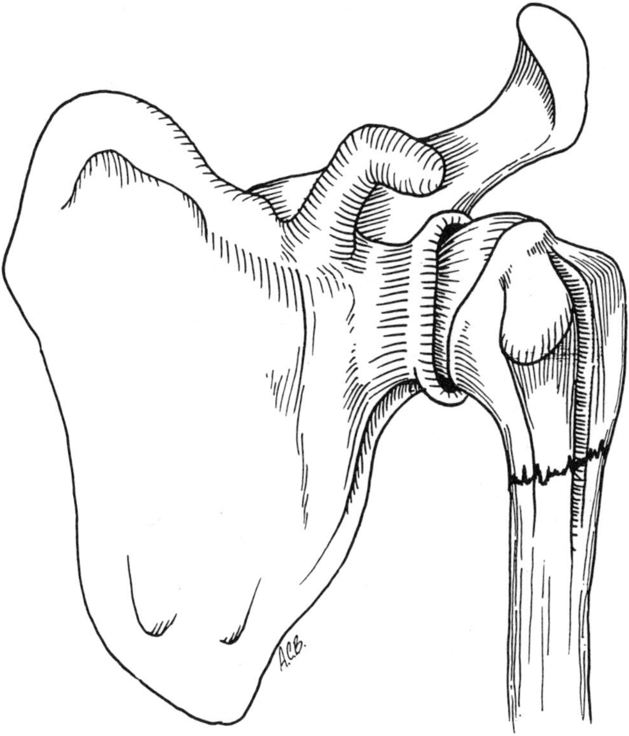
A.C.B.

FRACTURES OF THE PROXIMAL HUMERUS

(Neer Classification)

I. ONE-PART OR MINIMALLY DISPLACED FRACTURE WHERE NO SEGMENTS ARE DISPLACED BY 1.0 CM OR ANGULATED BY 45 DEGREES

II. TWO-PART FRACTURE WHERE ONE SEGMENT IS SIGNIFICANTLY DISPLACED BY 1.0 CM OR 45 DEGREES

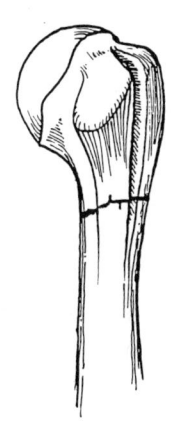

One Part Fracture

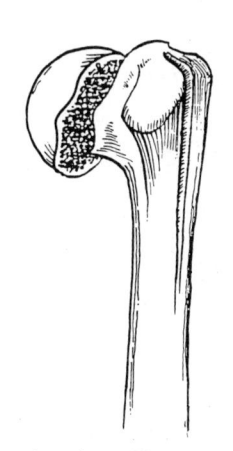

Two Part

Articular Segment Fracture

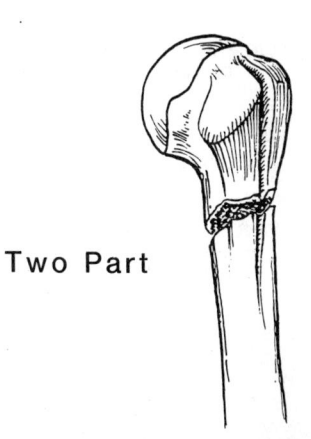

Humeral Shaft Fracture

FRACTURES OF THE PROXIMAL HUMERUS

(Neer Classification)

I. ONE-PART OR MINIMALLY DISPLACED FRACTURE WHERE NO SEGMENTS ARE DISPLACED BY 1.0 CM OR ANGULATED BY 45 DEGREES

II. TWO-PART FRACTURE WHERE ONE SEGMENT IS SIGNIFICANTLY DISPLACED BY 1.0 CM OR 45 DEGREES

III. THREE-PART FRACTURE WHERE TWO SEGMENTS ARE SIGNIFICANTLY DISPLACED BY 1.0 CM OR 45 DEGREES

IV. FOUR-PART FRACTURE WHERE ALL FOUR MAJOR SEGMENTS ARE DISPLACED BY 1.0 CM OR 45 DEGREES

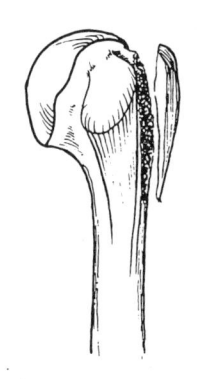

Two Part
Greater Tuberosity
Fracture

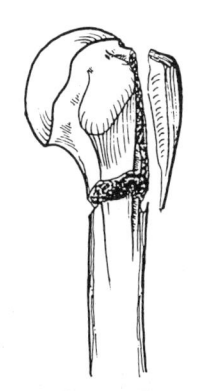

Three Part
Greater Tuberosity
and Shaft Fracture

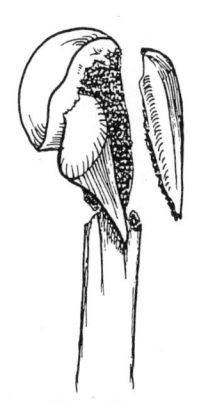

Four Part

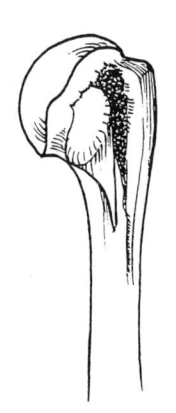

Two Part
Lesser Tuberosity
Fracture

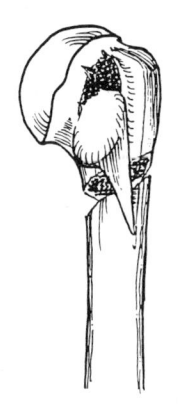

Three Part
Lesser Tuberosity
and Shaft Fracture

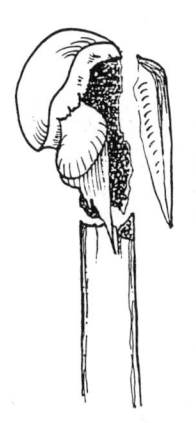

Four Part

FRACTURES OF THE PROXIMAL HUMERUS

(Neer Classification)

V. FRACTURE DISLOCATION

Fracture dislocations may be ANTERIOR or POSTERIOR and are also based on the four fracture segment classification.

Classification describes only displaced segments by 1.0 cm or 45 degree angulation.

Anterior Fracture Dislocations

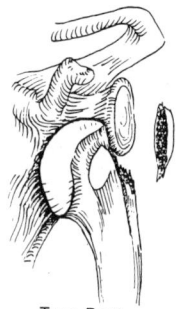

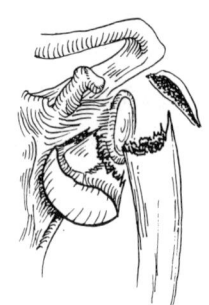

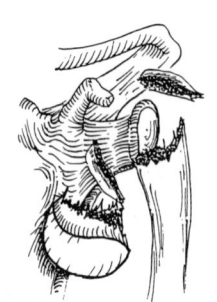

Two Part Three Part Four Part

Posterior Fracture Dislocations

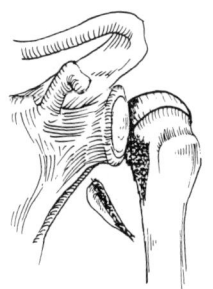

Two Part Three Part Four Part

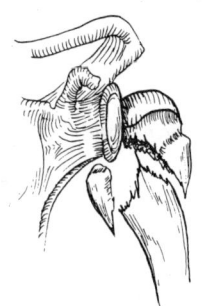

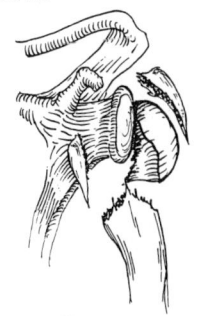

FRACTURES OF THE CLAVICLE

(Anatomic Location)

I.   INNER-THIRD - 5%[a]

II. MID-THIRD - 80%

III. DISTAL-THIRD OR INTERLIGAMENTOUS - 15%

DISTAL CLAVICLE FRACTURES are further subdivided on the next page.

[a] *Percentages indicate the frequency of fracture occurrence.*

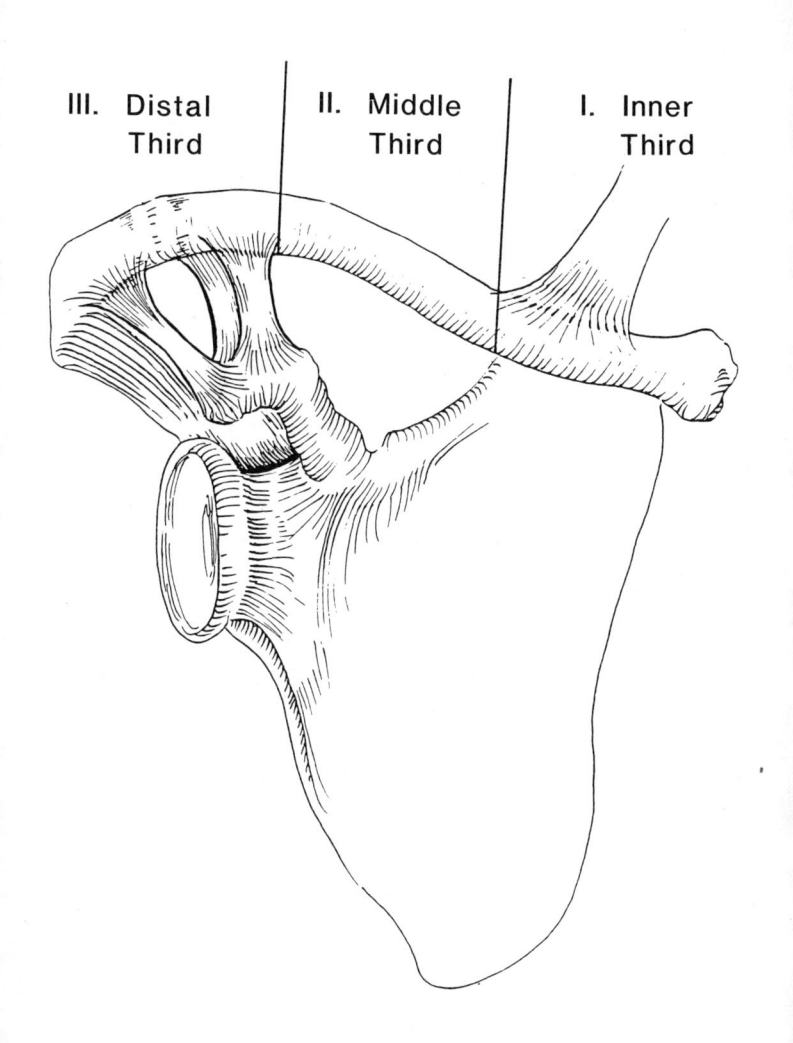

III. Distal Third   II. Middle Third   I. Inner Third

FRACTURES OF THE DISTAL CLAVICLE

(Neer Classification)

I. INTACT LIGAMENTS WITHOUT SIGNIFICANT DISPLACEMENT

II. DISPLACED INTERLIGAMENTOUS FRACTURE WHERE CORACOCLAVICULAR LIGAMENTS ARE DETACHED FROM THE MEDIAL SEGMENT AND TRAPEZOID LIGAMENTS REMAIN ATTACHED TO THE DISTAL SEGMENT

III. ARTICULAR SURFACE FRACTURES

I.

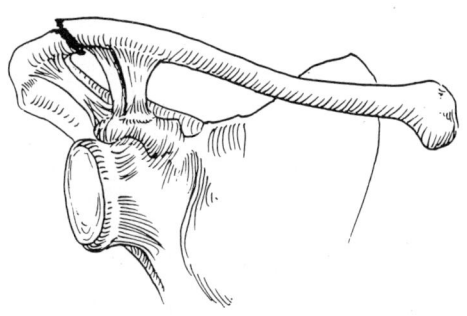

II.

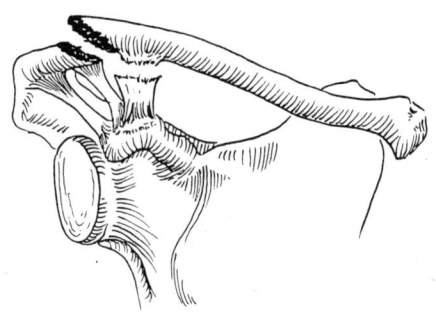

III.

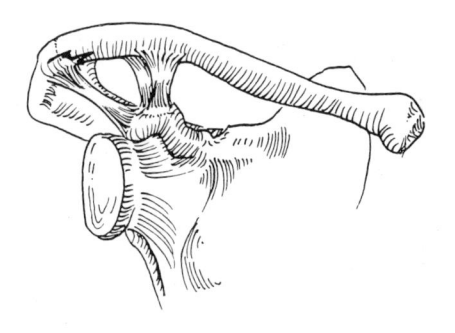

51

FRACTURES OF THE SCAPULA

(Anatomic Location)

I. NECK

II. ACROMIUM PROCESS

III. COROCOID PROCESS

IV. BODY

V. GLENOID RIM OR ARTICULAR SURFACE

VI. SPINOUS PROCESS

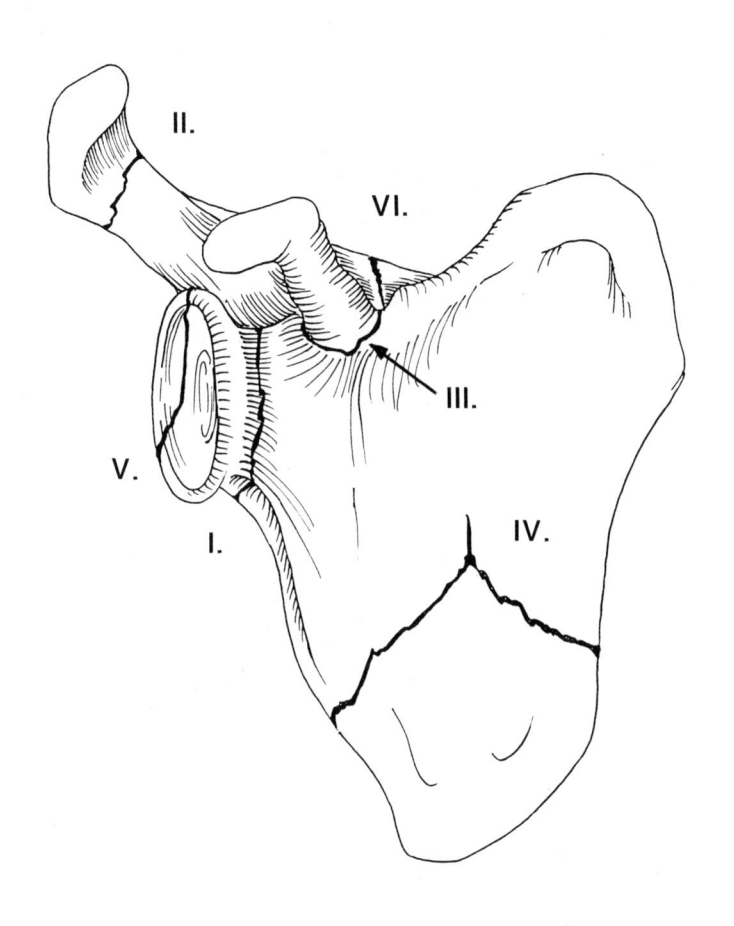

GLENOID FRACTURES

(Ideberg Classification)

I. FRACTURE OF THE ANTERIOR GLENOID MARGIN; ASSOCIATED WITH GLENOHUMERAL FRACTURE DISLOCATION

II. TRANSVERSE OR OBLIQUE FRACTURE THROUGH THE GLENOID FOSSA; MAY BE ASSOCIATED WITH INFERIOR HUMERAL HEAD SUBLUXATION OR DISLOCATION

III. OBLIQUE GLENOID FRACTURE THAT COURSES CEPHALAD TO THE MID PORTION OF THE SCAPULA

IV. HORIZONTAL FRACTURE THROUGH THE SCAPULA INVOLVING THE GLENOID FOSSA, NECK, AND BODY

V. HORIZONTAL FRACTURE COMBINED WITH TRANSVERSE COMPONENT INVOLVING THE ENTIRE SCAPULAR NECK OR JUST THE INFERIOR PORTION

Type I GLENOID FRACTURES are the most common.

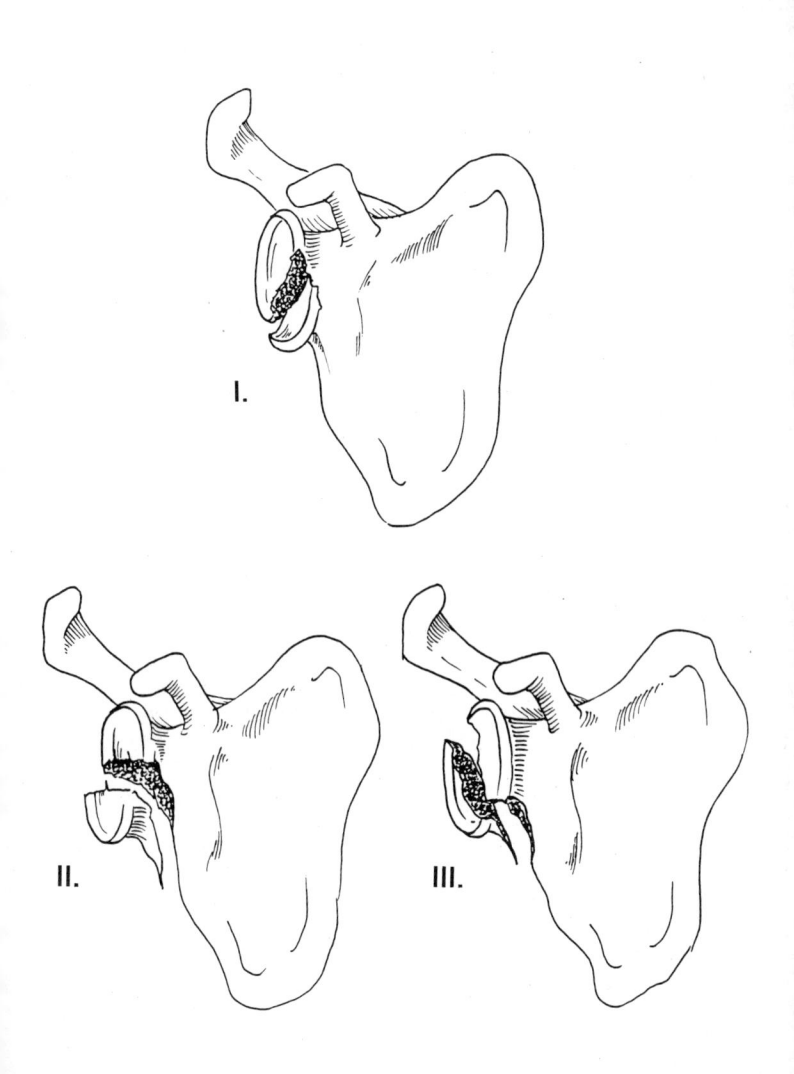

I.

II.

III.

GLENOID FRACTURES

(Ideberg Classification)

IV. HORIZONTAL FRACTURE THROUGH THE SCAPULA INVOLVING THE GLENOID FOSSA, NECK, AND BODY

V. HORIZONTAL FRACTURE COMBINED WITH TRANSVERSE COMPONENT INVOLVING THE ENTIRE SCAPULAR NECK OR JUST THE INFERIOR PORTION

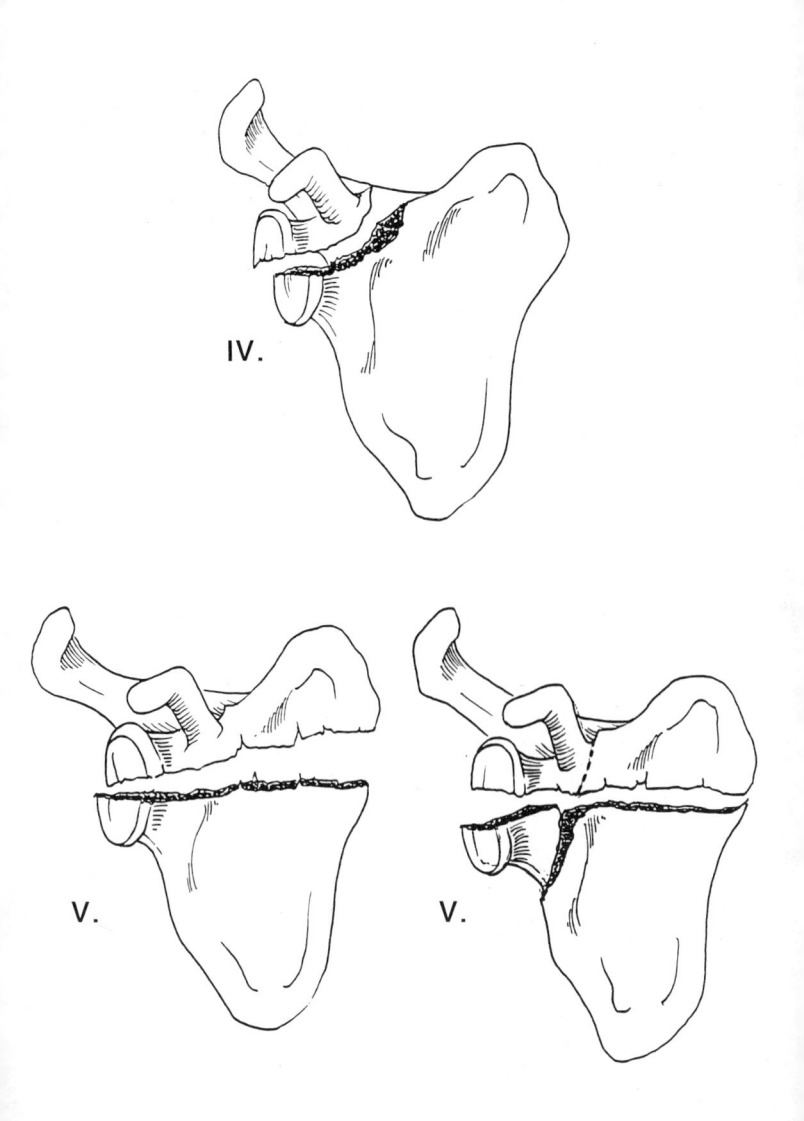

IV.

V. V.

57

SPINE

CLASSIFICATION OF CERVICAL SPINE INJURIES

(Harris Classification)

I. FLEXION
- A. ANTERIOR SUBLUXATION
- B. BILATERAL INTERFACETAL DISLOCATION
- C. SIMPLE WEDGE (COMPRESSION) FRACTURE
- D. CLAY-SHOVELER (COAL-SHOVELER) FRACTURE
- E. FLEXION TEARDROP FRACTURE

II. FLEXION-ROTATION: UNILATERAL INTERFACETAL DISLOCATION

III. EXTENSION-ROTATION: PILLAR FRACTURE

IV. VERTICAL COMPRESSION
- A. JEFFERSON BURST FRACTURE OF ATLAS
- B. BURST FRACTURE

V. HYPEREXTENSION
- A. HYPEREXTENSION DISLOCATION
- B. AVULSION FRACTURE OF ANTERIOR ARCH OF THE ATLAS
- C. EXTENSION TEARDROP FRACTURE OF THE AXIS
- D. FRACTURE OF THE POSTERIOR ARCH OF THE ATLAS
- E. LAMINAR FRACTURE
- F. TRAUMATIC SPONDYLOLISTHESIS (HANGMAN'S FRACTURE)
- G. HYPEREXTENSION FRACTURE DISLOCATION

VI. LATERAL FLEXION: UNCINATE PROCESS FRACTURE

VII. DIVERSE, OR IMPRECISELY UNDERSTOOD, MECHANISMS
- A. ATLANTA-OCCIPITAL DISASSOCIATION
- B. ODONTOID FRACTURES

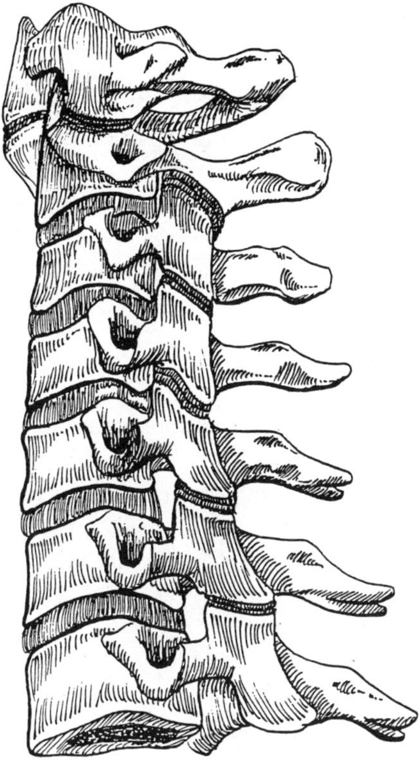

CLASSIFICATION OF CERVICAL SPINE INJURIES

(Harris Classification)

I. FLEXION

    A. ANTERIOR SUBLUXATION

    B. BILATERAL INTERFACETAL DISLOCATION

    C. SIMPLE WEDGE (COMPRESSION) FRACTURE

    D. CLAY-SHOVELER (COAL-SHOVELER) FRACTURE

    E. FLEXION TEARDROP FRACTURE

Additional descriptions of CLAY-SHOVELER FRACTURE in the EPONYM SECTION.

I. A.

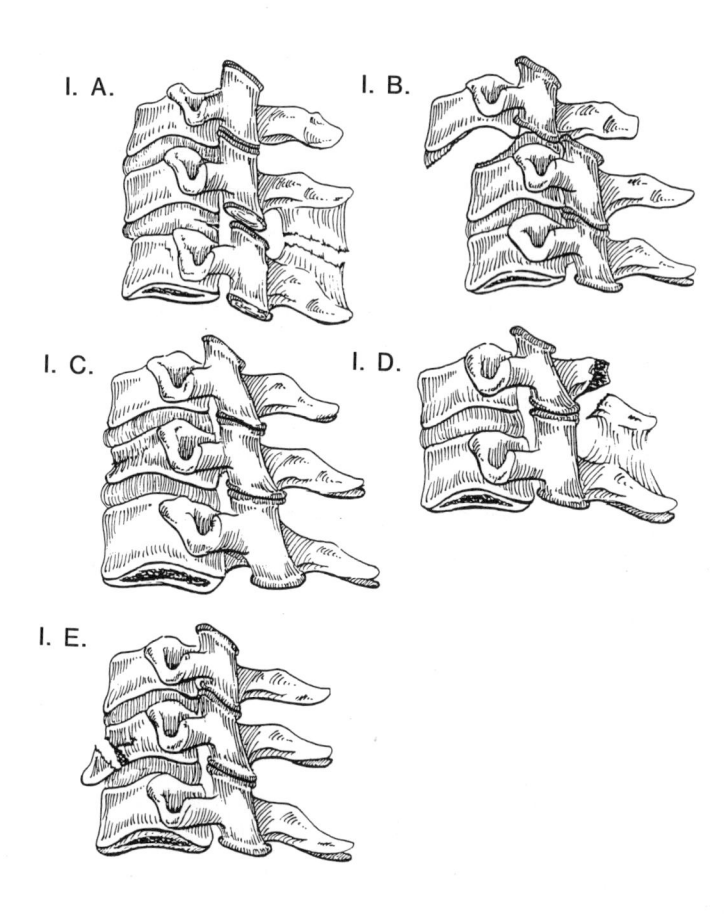

I. B.

I. C.

I. D.

I. E.

CLASSIFICATION OF CERVICAL SPINE INJURIES

(Harris Classification)

II. FLEXION-ROTATION: UNILATERAL INTERFACETAL DISLOCATION

III. EXTENSION-ROTATION: PILLAR FRACTURE

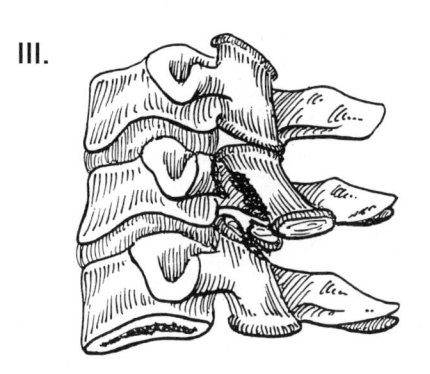

II.

III.

CLASSIFICATION OF CERVICAL SPINE INJURIES

(Harris Classification)

IV. VERTICAL COMPRESSION

    A. JEFFERSON BURST FRACTURE OF ATLAS

    B. BURST FRACTURE

IV. A.

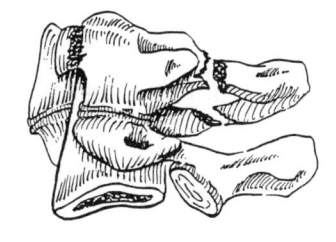

Lateral View 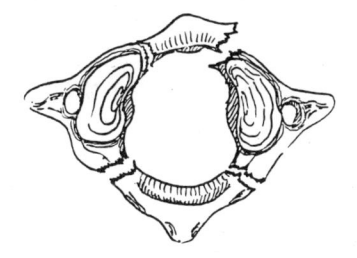   Axial View

IV. B.

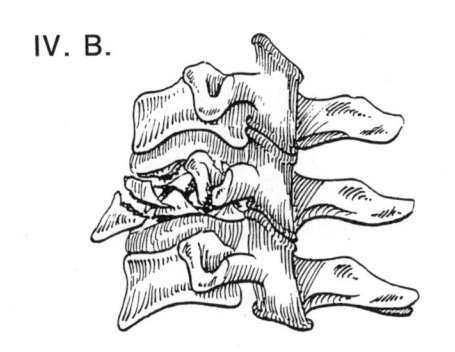

CLASSIFICATION OF CERVICAL SPINE INJURIES

(Harris Classification)

V. HYPEREXTENSION

    A. HYPEREXTENSION DISLOCATION

    B. AVULSION FRACTURE OF ANTERIOR ARCH OF THE ATLAS

    C. EXTENSION TEARDROP FRACTURE OF THE AXIS

    D. FRACTURE OF THE POSTERIOR ARCH OF THE ATLAS

    E. LAMINAR FRACTURE

    F. TRAUMATIC SPONDYLOLISTHESIS (HANGMAN'S FRACTURE)

    G. HYPERXTENSION FRACTURE DISLOCATION

V. A.

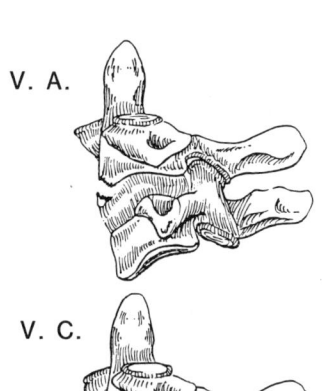

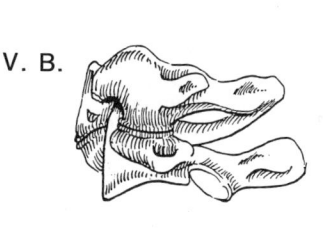

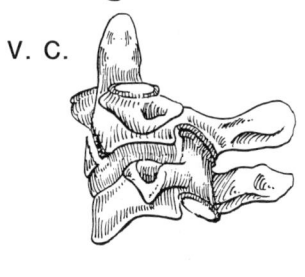

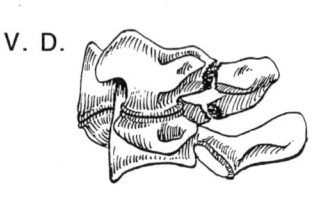

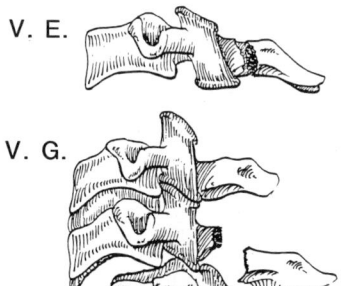

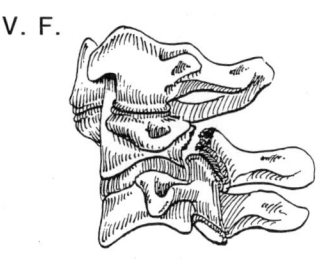

V. B.

V. C.

V. D.

V. E.

V. F.

V. G.

CLASSIFICATION OF CERVICAL SPINE INJURIES

(Harris Classification)

VI. LATERAL FLEXION: UNCINATE PROCESS FRACTURE

VII. DIVERSE, OR IMPRECISELY UNDERSTOOD, MECHANISMS

    A. ATLANTA-OCCIPITAL DISASSOCIATION

    B. ODONTOID FRACTURES

ODONTOID FRACTURE classification is located on the next page.

VI.

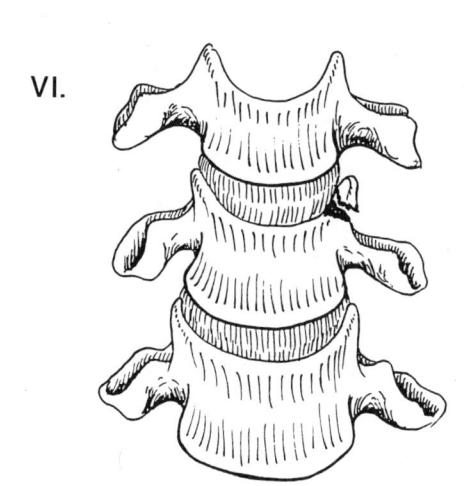

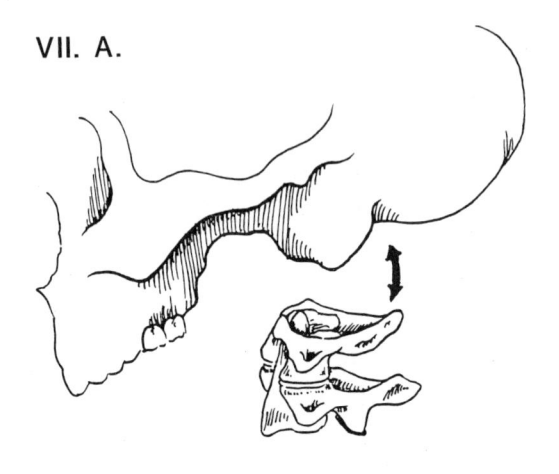

VII. A.

FRACTURES OF THE ODONTOID PROCESS

(Anderson and D'Alonzo Classification)

I. OBLIQUE FRACTURE THROUGH THE SUPERIOR PART OF THE ODONTOID

II. FRACTURE AT THE JUNCTION OF THE ODONTOID PROCESS AND THE AXIS

III. FRACTURE EXTENDS INTO THE BODY OF THE AXIS

ODONTOID FRACTURES may be further classified as DISPLACED or NONDISPLACED.

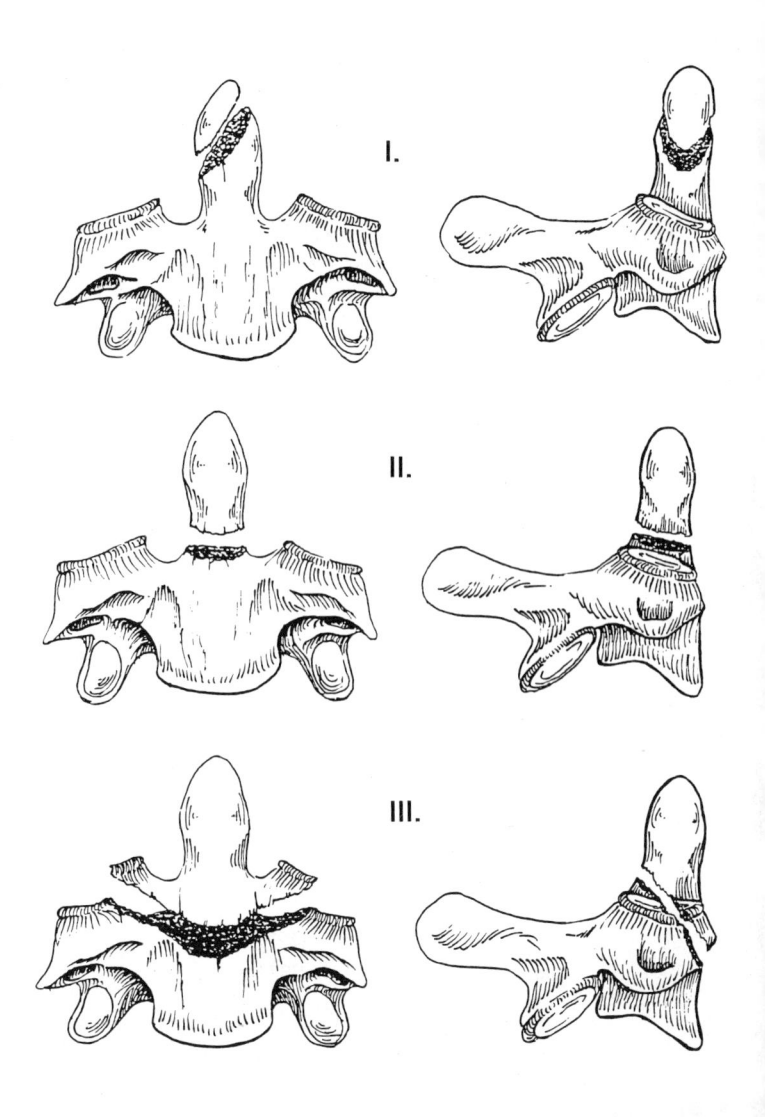

I.

II.

III.

73

THORACOLUMBAR SPINAL INJURY CLASSIFICATION

(Denis Classification)

I. MINOR SPINAL INJURIES

    A. ARTICULAR PROCESS FRACTURE

    B. TRANSVERSE PROCESS FRACTURE

    C. SPINOUS PROCESS FRACTURE

    D. PARS INTERARTICULARIS FRACTURE

II. MAJOR SPINAL INJURIES

    A. COMPRESSION FRACTURE

    B. BURST FRACTURES

    C. FRACTURE DISLOCATIONS

    D. SEAT-BELT TYPE SPINAL INJURIES

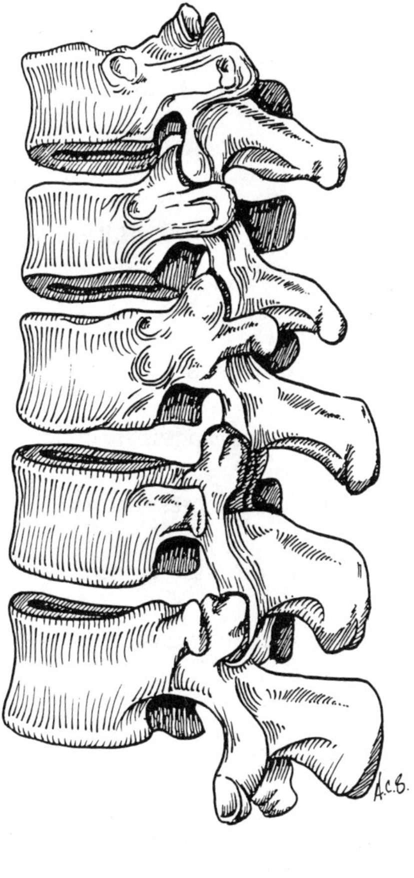
A.C.B.

THORACOLUMBAR SPINAL INJURY CLASSIFICATION

(Denis Classification)

I. MINOR SPINAL INJURIES

    A. TRANSVERSE PROCESS FRACTURE

    B. ARTICULAR PROCESS FRACTURE

    C. SPINOUS PROCESS FRACTURE

    D. PARS INTERARTICULARIS FRACTURE

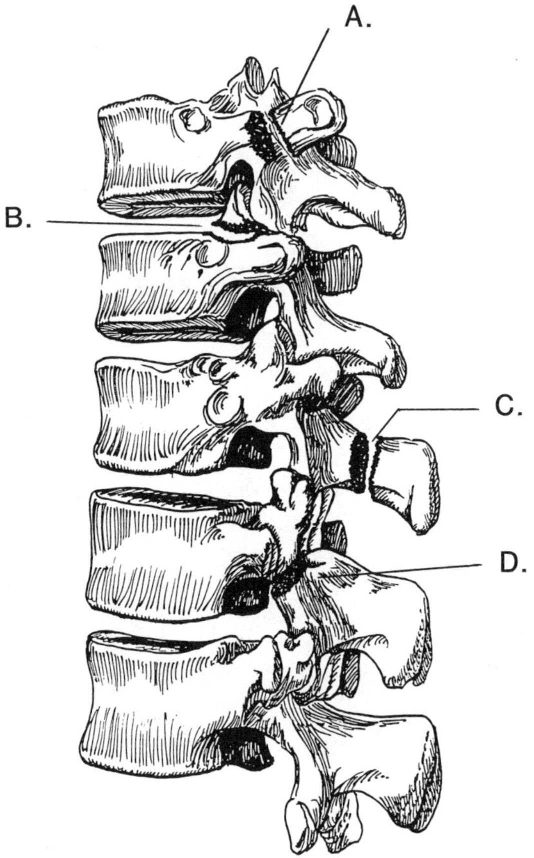
A.
B.
C.
D.

THORACOLUMBAR SPINAL INJURY CLASSIFICATION

(Denis Classification)

II. MAJOR SPINAL INJURIES

    A. COMPRESSION FRACTURE

    B. BURST FRACTURES

BURST FRACTURES disrupt middle spinal segment and retropulse bone fragments toward the spinal canal.

II. A.

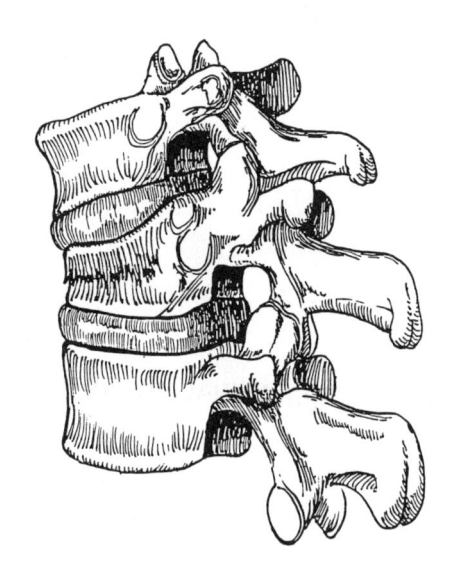

II. B.

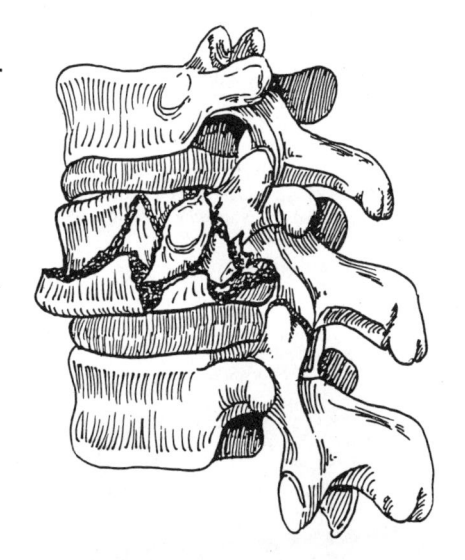

THORACOLUMBAR SPINAL INJURY CLASSIFICATION

(Denis Classification)

II. MAJOR SPINAL INJURIES

    C. FRACTURE DISLOCATIONS

    D. SEAT-BELT TYPE SPINAL INJURIES

SEAT-BELT TYPE SPINAL INJURIES may be through bone, ligaments or a combination. Mechanism of injury is usually a flexion distraction type force.

II. C.

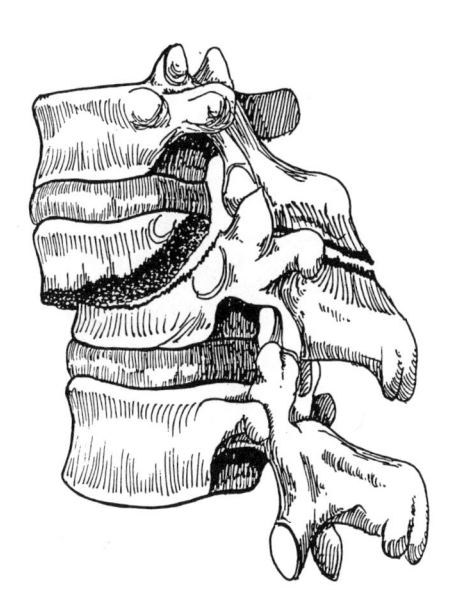

II. D.

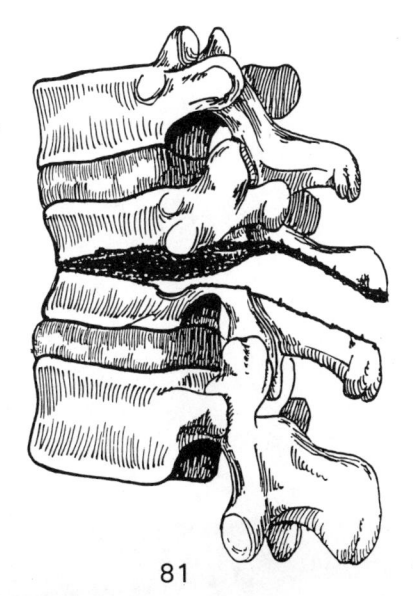

PELVIS and ACETABULUM

CLASSIFICATION OF PELVIC DISRUPTION

(Tile Classification)

TYPE A. STABLE

    A1. FRACTURES OF THE PELVIS NOT INVOLVING THE RING

    A2. STABLE, MINIMALLY DISPLACED FRACTURES OF THE RING

TYPE B. ROTATIONALLY UNSTABLE, VERTICALLY STABLE

    B1. OPEN BOOK

    B2. LATERAL COMPRESSION: IPSILATERAL

    B3. LATERAL COMPRESSION: CONTRALATERAL (BUCKET HANDLE)

TYPE C. ROTATIONALLY AND VERTICALLY UNSTABLE

    C1. UNILATERAL

    C2. BILATERAL

    C3. ASSOCIATED WITH ACETABULAR FRACTURE

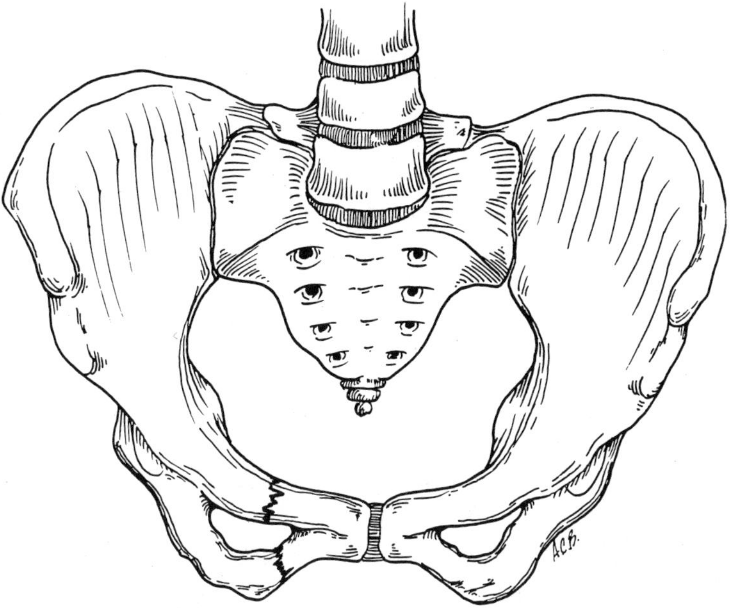
ACB.

CLASSIFICATION OF PELVIC DISRUPTION

(Tile Classification)

TYPE A.   STABLE

  A1.   FRACTURES OF THE PELVIS NOT INVOLVING THE RING

  A2.   STABLE, MINIMALLY DISPLACED FRACTURES OF THE RING

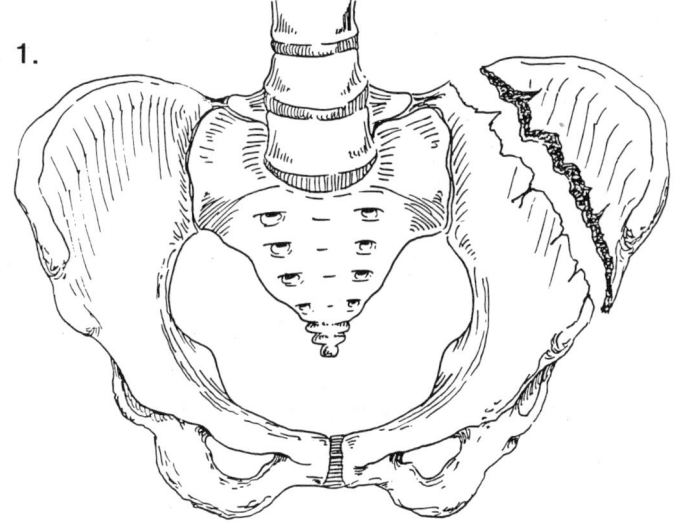

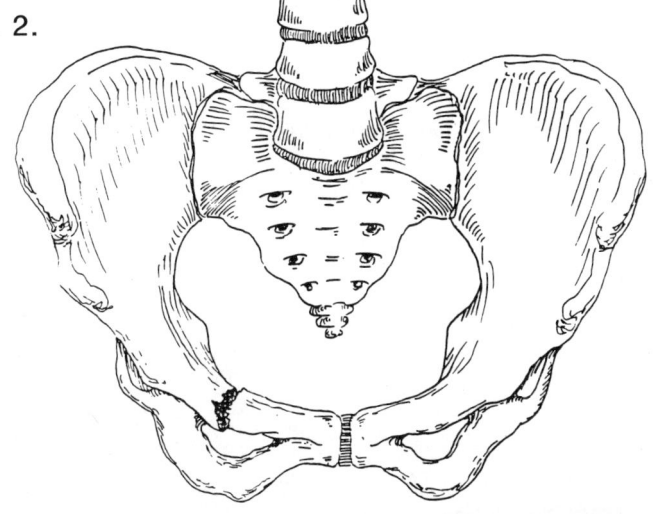

A. 1.

A. 2.

CLASSIFICATION OF PELVIC DISRUPTION

(Tile Classification)

TYPE B.   ROTATIONALLY UNSTABLE, VERTICALLY STABLE

   B1.   OPEN BOOK

   B2.   LATERAL COMPRESSION: IPSILATERAL

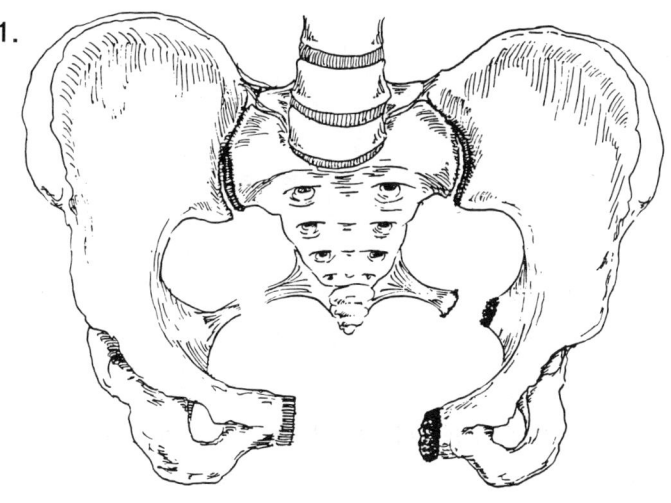

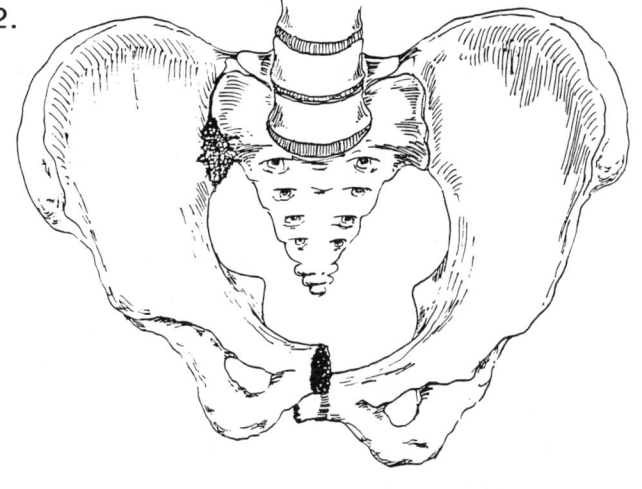

B. 1.

B. 2.

CLASSIFICATION OF PELVIC DISRUPTION

(Tile Classification)

TYPE B.   ROTATIONALLY UNSTABLE, VERTICALLY STABLE

     B3.   LATERAL COMPRESSION: CONTRALATERAL (BUCKET HANDLE)

B. 3.

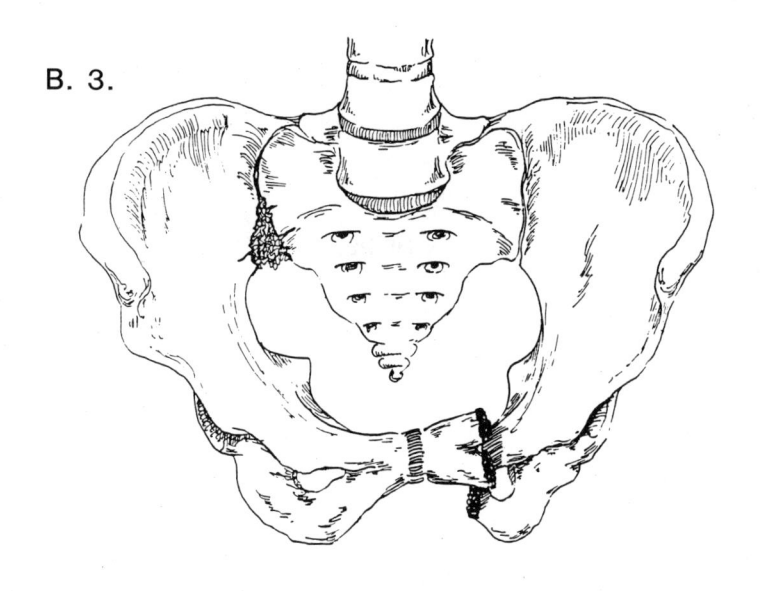

CLASSIFICATION OF PELVIC DISRUPTION

(Tile Classification)

TYPE C. ROTATIONALLY AND VERTICALLY UNSTABLE

    C1. UNILATERAL

    C2. BILATERAL

    C3. ASSOCIATED WITH ACETABULAR FRACTURE

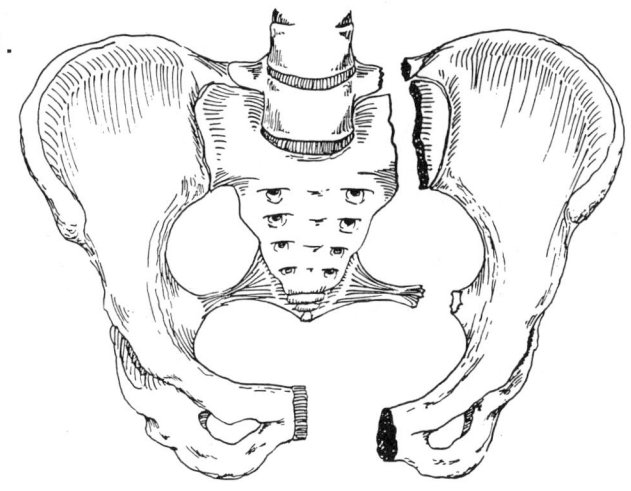

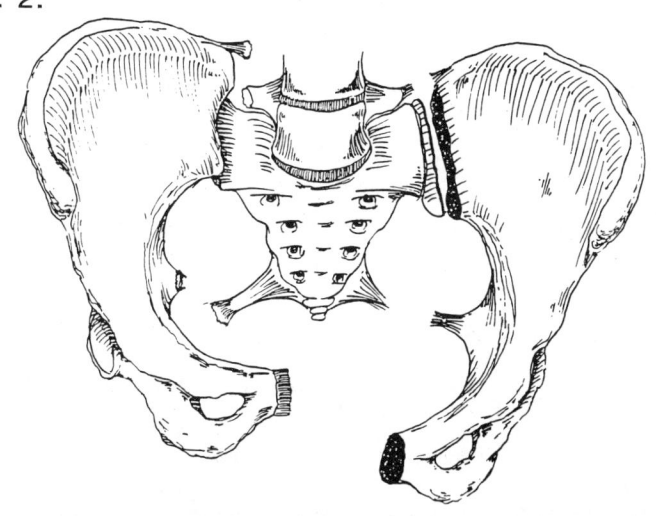

C. 1.

C. 2.

CLASSIFICATION OF ACETABULUM FRACTURES

(Tile Classification)

UNDISPLACED

DISPLACED

- TYPE I. POSTERIOR TYPES WITH OR WITHOUT POSTERIOR DISLOCATION
  - A. POSTERIOR COLUMN
  - B. POSTERIOR WALL
    1. ASSOCIATED WITH POSTERIOR COLUMN
    2. ASSOCIATED WITH TRANSVERSE FRACTURES
- TYPE II. ANTERIOR TYPES WITH OR WITHOUT ANTERIOR DISLOCATIONS
  - A. ANTERIOR COLUMN
  - B. ANTERIOR WALL
  - C. ASSOCIATED WITH ANTERIOR WALL, ANTERIOR COLUMN, AND/OR TRANSVERSE FRACTURES
- TYPE III. TRANSVERSE TYPES WITH OR WITHOUT CENTRAL DISLOCATION
  - A. PURE TRANSVERSE
  - B. T-FRACTURES
  - C. ASSOCIATED TRANSVERSE AND ACETABULAR WALL FRACTURES
  - D. DOUBLE COLUMN FRACTURES

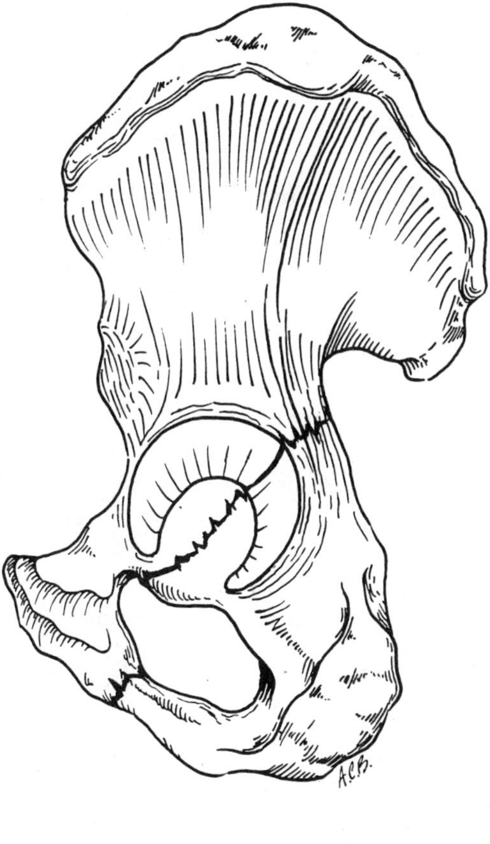
A.C.B.

CLASSIFICATION OF ACETABULUM FRACTURES

(Tile Classification)

DISPLACED

    TYPE I.   POSTERIOR TYPES WITH OR WITHOUT POSTERIOR DISLOCATION

        A.   POSTERIOR COLUMN

        B.   POSTERIOR WALL

            1.   ASSOCIATED WITH POSTERIOR COLUMN

            2.   ASSOCIATED WITH TRANSVERSE FRACTURES

I. A.

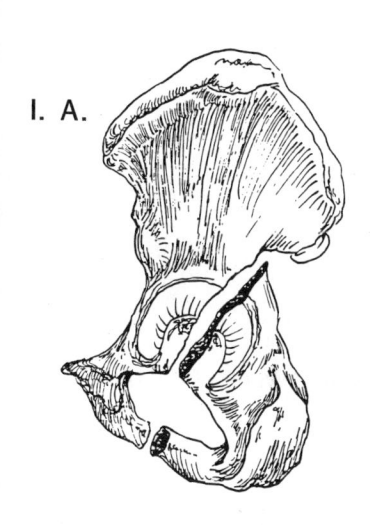

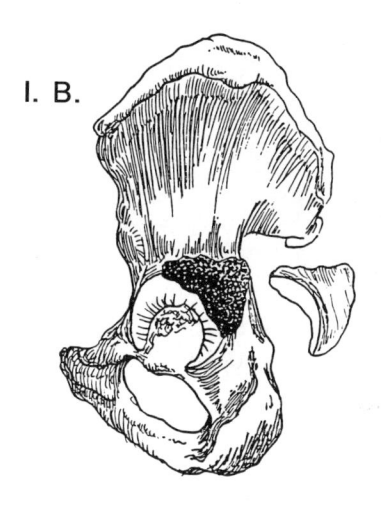

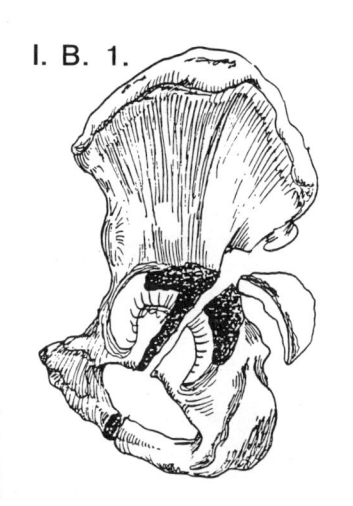

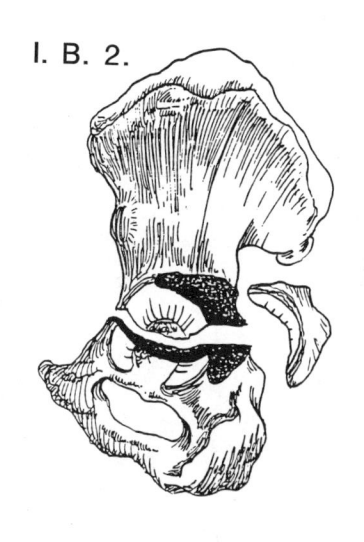

I. B.

I. B. 1.

I. B. 2.

CLASSIFICATION OF ACETABULUM FRACTURES

(Tile Classification)

DISPLACED

    TYPE II.   ANTERIOR TYPES WITH OR WITHOUT ANTERIOR DISLOCATIONS

        A.   ANTERIOR COLUMN

        B.   ANTERIOR WALL

        C.   ASSOCIATED WITH ANTERIOR WALL, ANTERIOR COLUMN, AND/OR TRANSVERSE FRACTURES

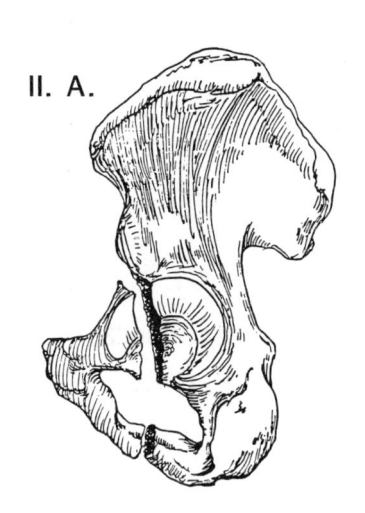

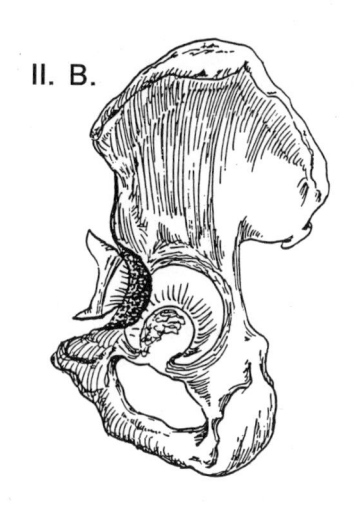

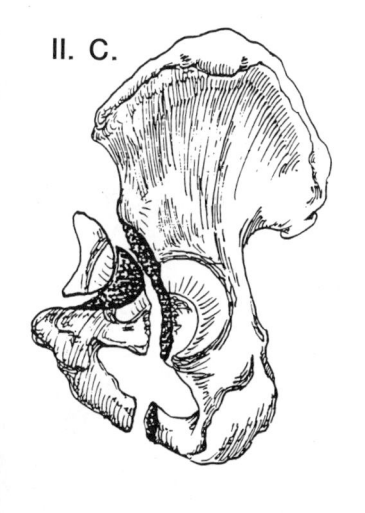

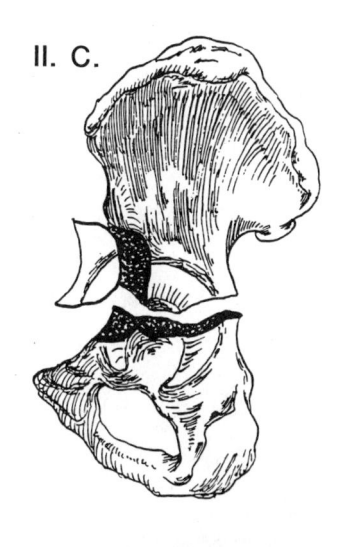

II. A.

II. B.

II. C.

II. C.

CLASSIFICATION OF ACETABULUM FRACTURES

(Tile Classification)

DISPLACED

- TYPE III. TRANSVERSE TYPES WITH OR WITHOUT CENTRAL DISLOCATION

    A. PURE TRANSVERSE

    B. T-FRACTURES

    C. ASSOCIATED TRANSVERSE AND ACETABULAR WALL FRACTURES

    D. DOUBLE COLUMN FRACTURES

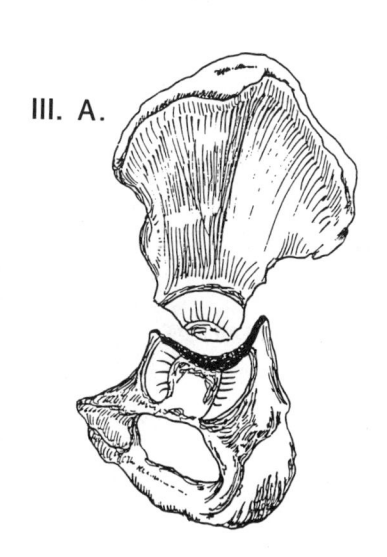

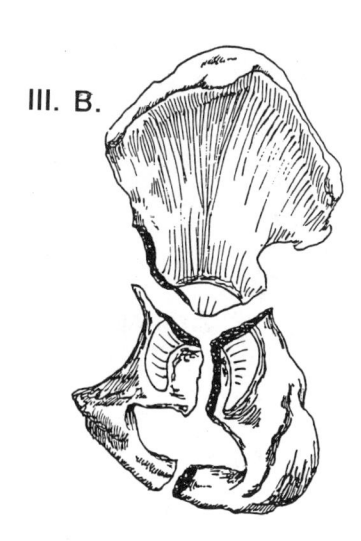

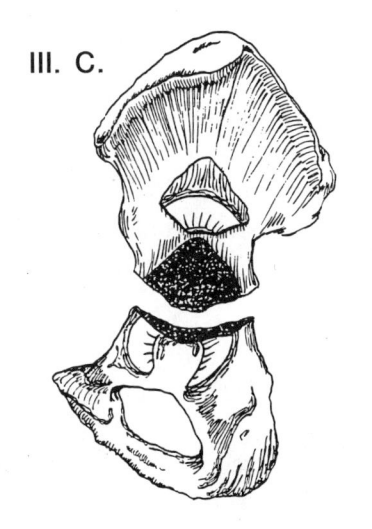

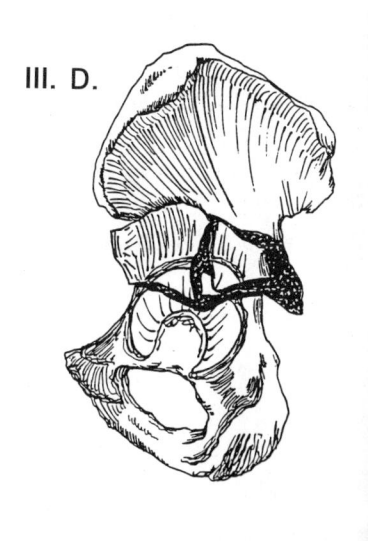

III. A.

III. B.

III. C.

III. D.

SACRAL FRACTURE CLASSIFICATION

(Denis Classification)

I. FRACTURE THROUGH SACRAL ALA WITHOUT DAMAGE TO THE CENTRAL CANAL OR SACRAL FORAMINA

II. FRACTURE INVOLVING THE SACRAL FORAMINA BUT SPARING THE CENTRAL CANAL. FRACTURE MAY ALSO INVOLVE THE ALAR ZONE

III. FRACTURE INVOLVING THE CENTRAL SACRAL CANAL. FRACTURE MAY ALSO INVOLVE FORAMINA AND ALAR ZONES

Zone II fractures are frequently associated with sciatica and nerve root injury.

Zone III fractures are frequently associated with loss of sphincter function and saddle anesthesia.

I. II. III.

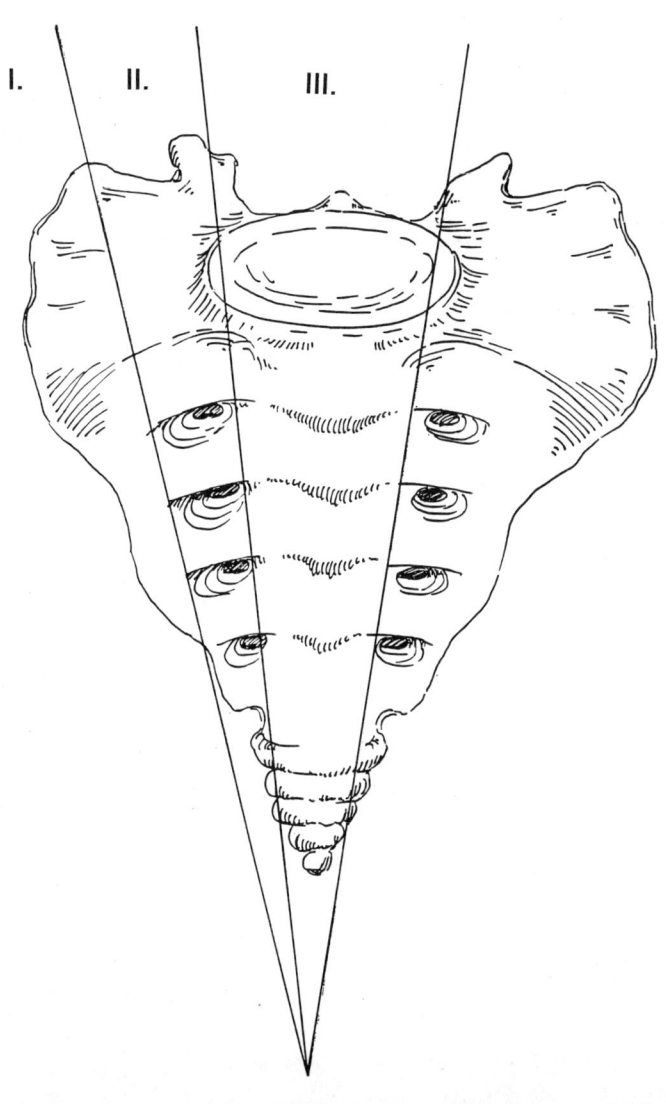

LOWER EXTREMITY

CLASSIFICATION OF HIP FRACTURES

(Anatomic Classification)

I. FEMORAL NECK - INTRACAPSULAR FRACTURES
   (Garden Classification)

II. INTERTROCHANTERIC - EXTRACAPSULAR FRACTURE
   (Kyle Classification)

III. SUBTROCHANTERIC
   (Seinsheimer Classification)

I.
II.
III.

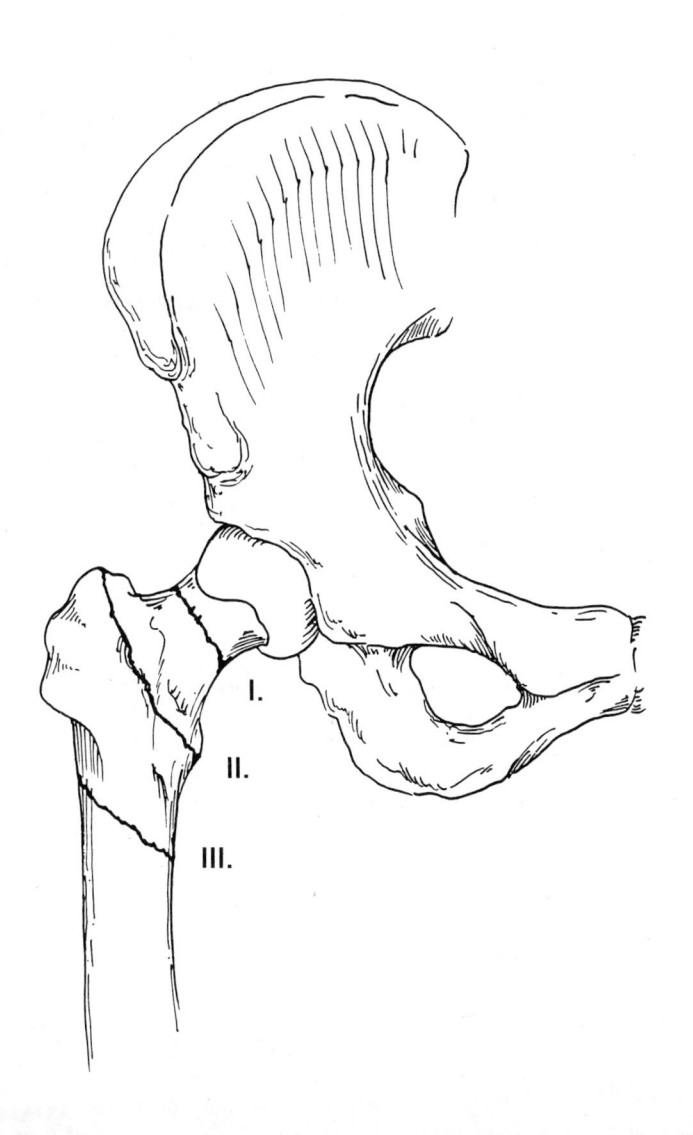

107

FRACTURES OF THE FEMORAL NECK

(Garden Classification)

I. INCOMPLETE OR IMPACTED FRACTURE

II. COMPLETE FRACTURE WITHOUT DISPLACEMENT

III. COMPLETE FRACTURE WITH PARTIAL DISPLACEMENT
 (HIP CAPSULE USUALLY PARTIALLY INTACT)

IV. COMPLETE FRACTURE WITH FULL DISPLACEMENT
 (HIP CAPSULE USUALLY COMPLETELY DISRUPTED)

Greater fracture displacement increases the incidence of avascular necrosis.

Type I femoral neck fractures may present with coxa valgus, while type III fractures demonstrate coxa varus.

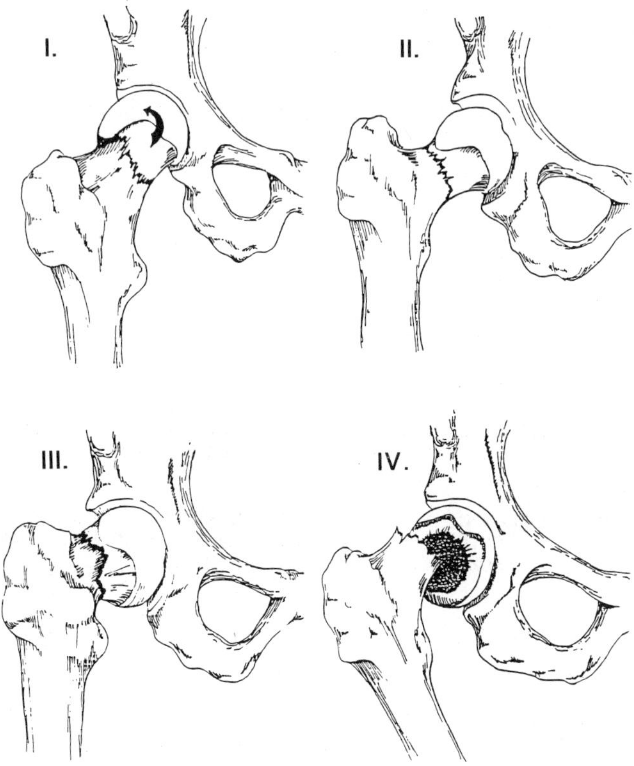
I.
II.
III.
IV.

INTERTROCHANTERIC HIP FRACTURES

(Kyle Classification)

I. NONDISPLACED STABLE INTERTROCHANTERIC FRACTURE WITHOUT COMMINUTION

II. DISPLACED STABLE INTERTROCHANTERIC FRACTURE WITH MINIMAL COMMINUTION

III. DISPLACED UNSTABLE INTERTROCHANTERIC FRACTURE WITH EXTENSIVE POSTERIOR MEDIAL COMMINUTION

IV. DISPLACED UNSTABLE INTERTROCHANTERIC FRACTURE WITH EXTENSIVE POSTERIOR MEDIAL COMMINUTION AND A SUBTROCHANTERIC COMPONENT

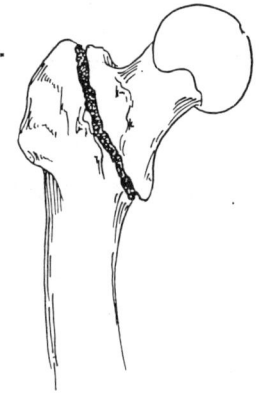

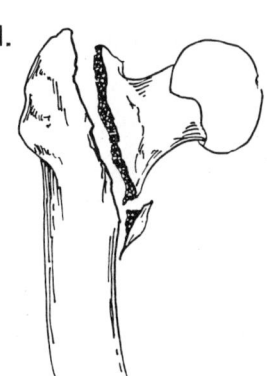

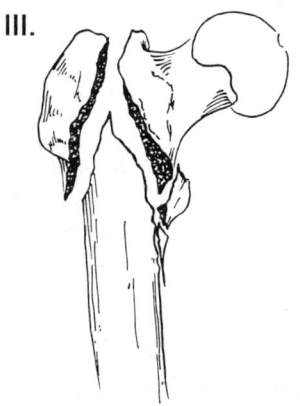

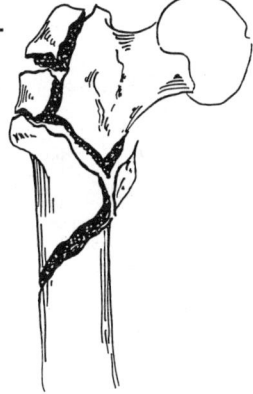

I.

II.

III.

IV.

SUBTROCHANTERIC FRACTURES OF THE FEMUR

(Seinsheimer Classification)

I. NONDISPLACED FRACTURE WITH LESS THAN 2 MM OF DISPLACEMENT

II. TWO-PART FRACTURES

    IIA. TWO-PART TRANSVERSE FEMORAL FRACTURE

    IIB. TWO-PART SPIRAL FRACTURE WITH LESSER TROCHANTER ATTACHED TO PROXIMAL FRAGMENT

    IIC. TWO-PART SPIRAL FRACTURE WITH LESSER TROCHANTER ATTACHED TO DISTAL FRAGMENT

III. THREE-PART FRACTURES

    IIIA. THREE-PART SPIRAL FRACTURE IN WHICH THE LESSER TROCHANTER IS PART OF THE THIRD FRAGMENT

    IIIB. THREE-PART SPIRAL FRACTURE IN WHICH THE THIRD PART IS A BUTTERFLY FRAGMENT

IV. COMMINUTED FRACTURE WITH FOUR OR MORE FRAGMENTS

V. SUBTROCHANTERIC - INTERTROCHANTERIC FRACTURE, ANY SUBTROCHANTERIC FRACTURE WITH EXTENSION THROUGH THE GREATER TROCHANTER

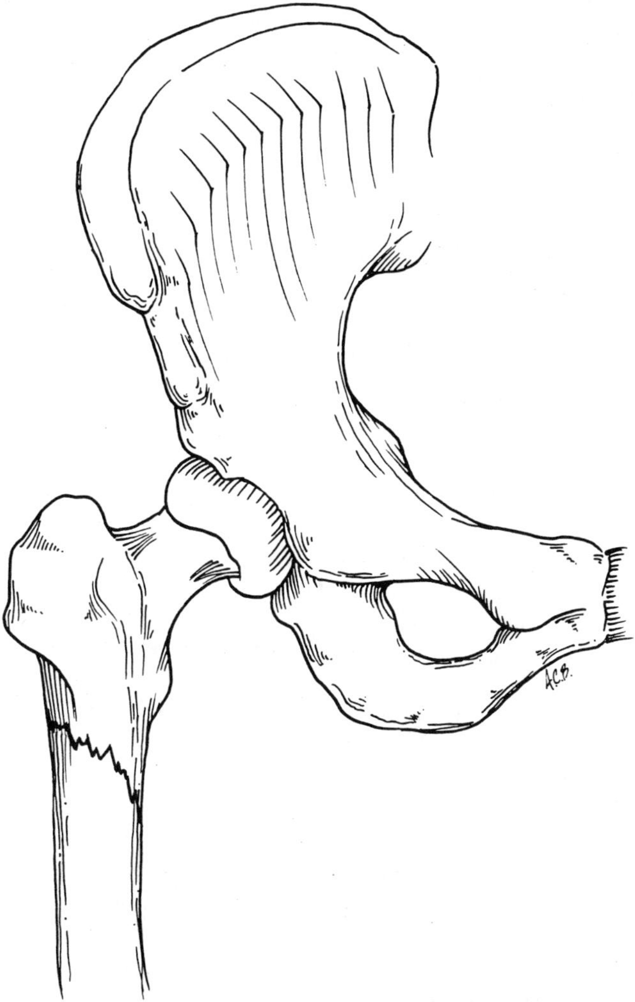
A.C.B.

SUBTROCHANTERIC FRACTURES OF THE FEMUR

(Seinsheimer Classification)

I. NONDISPLACED FRACTURE WITH LESS THAN 2 MM OF DISPLACEMENT

II. TWO-PART FRACTURES

   IIA. TWO-PART TRANSVERSE FEMORAL FRACTURE

   IIB. TWO-PART SPIRAL FRACTURE WITH LESSER TROCHANTER ATTACHED TO PROXIMAL FRAGMENT

   IIC. TWO-PART SPIRAL FRACTURE WITH LESSER TROCHANTER ATTACHED TO DISTAL FRAGMENT

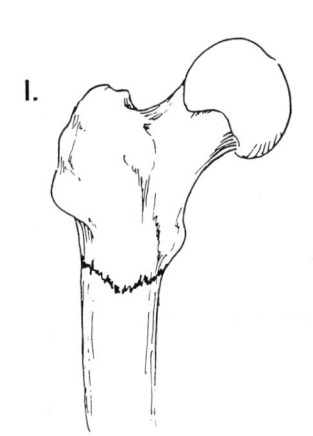

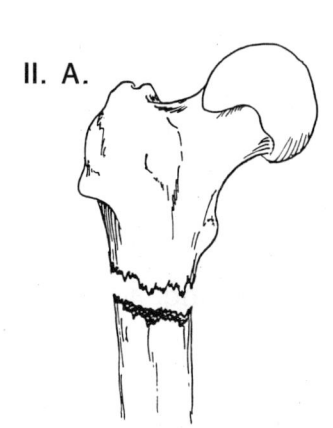

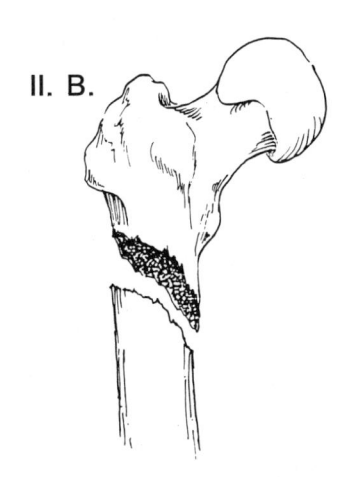

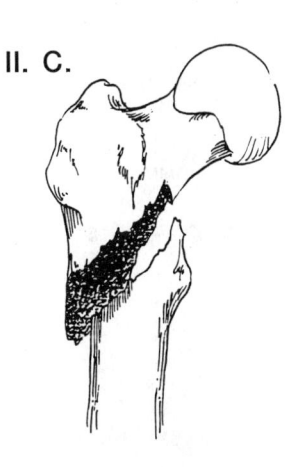

I.

II. A.

II. B.

II. C.

115

SUBTROCHANTERIC FRACTURES OF THE FEMUR

(Seinsheimer Classification)

III. THREE-PART FRACTURES

    IIIA. THREE-PART SPIRAL FRACTURE IN WHICH THE LESSER TROCHANTER IS PART OF THE THIRD FRAGMENT

    IIIB. THREE-PART SPIRAL FRACTURE IN WHICH THE THIRD PART IS A BUTTERFLY FRAGMENT

IV. COMMINUTED FRACTURE WITH FOUR OR MORE FRAGMENTS

V. SUBTROCHANTERIC - INTERTROCHANTERIC FRACTURE

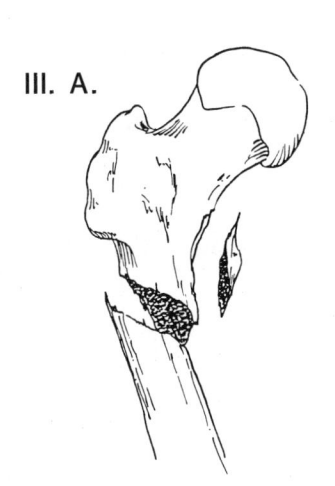

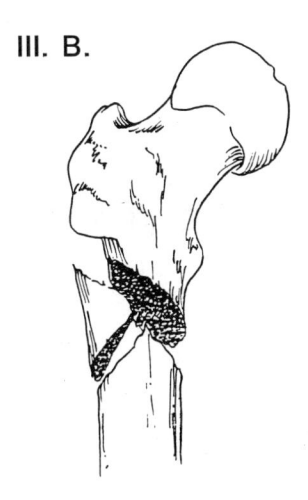

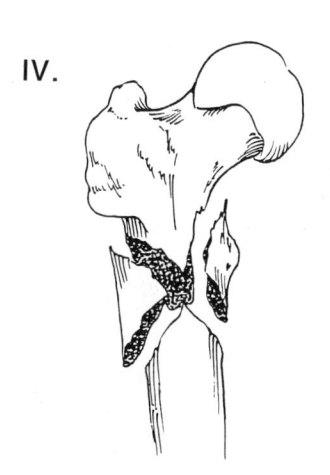

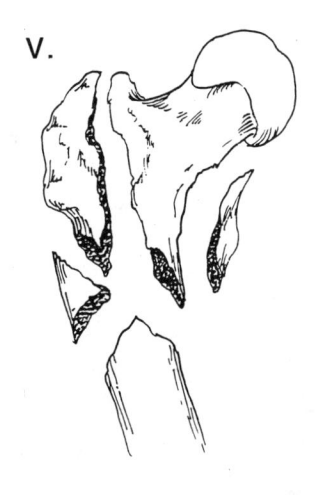

III. A.

III. B.

IV.

V.

FEMORAL SHAFT FRACTURES

(Winquist Classification of Comminution)

I. FEMORAL SHAFT FRACTURE WITH VERY SMALL BUTTERFLY FRAGMENT (25% OR LESS OF THE WIDTH OF THE BONE)

II. COMMINUTED FEMORAL SHAFT FRACTURE WITH BUTTERFLY FRAGMENT 50% OR LESS OF THE WIDTH OF THE BONE

III. COMMINUTED FRACTURE WITH LARGE BUTTERFLY SEGMENT GREATER THAN 50% OF THE WIDTH OF THE BONE

IV. SEVERE COMMINUTION OF AN ENTIRE SEGMENT OF BONE

V. FEMORAL SHAFT FRACTURE WITH SEGMENTAL BONE LOSS

Increasing comminution decreases inherent stability to rotation, shortening, and angulation.

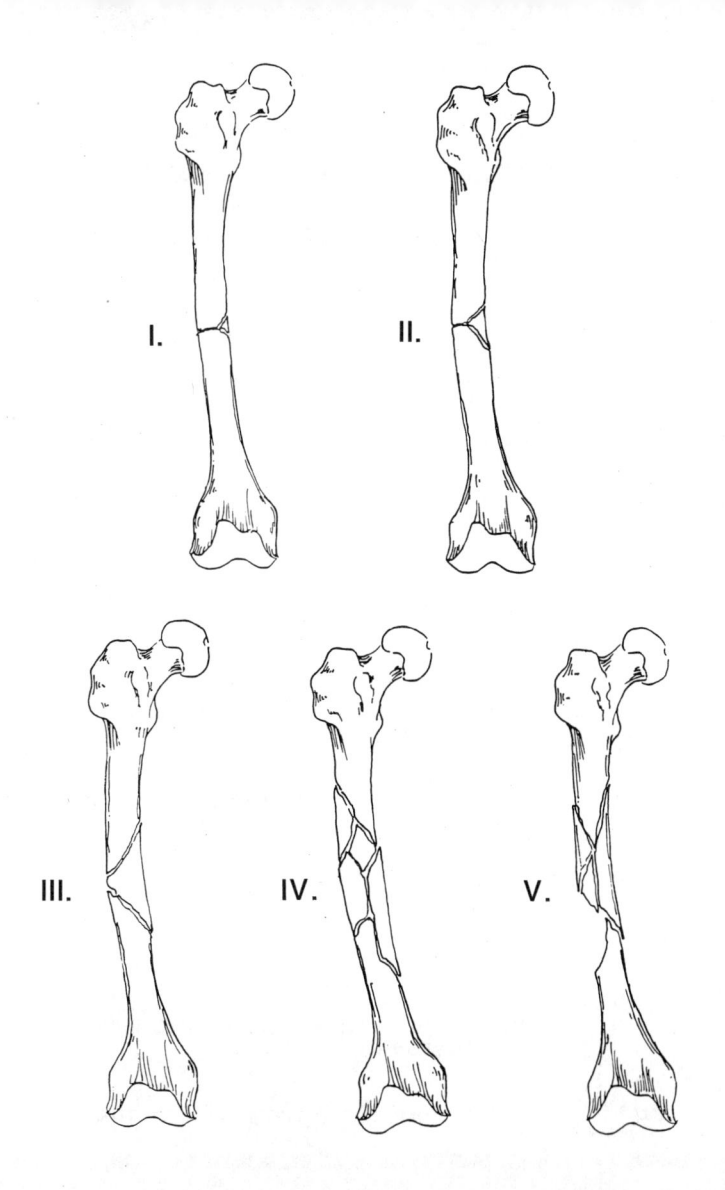

I.   II.

III.   IV.   V.

SUPRACONDYLAR FEMORAL FRACTURES

(AO Classification)

A. EXTRA-ARTICULAR

    A1. AVULSION OF THE MEDIAL OR LATERAL EPICONDYLE

    A2. SIMPLE SUPRACONDYLAR

    A3. COMMINUTED SUPRACONDYLAR

B. UNICONDYLAR

    B1. MEDIAL OR LATERAL CONDYLE

    B2. CONDYLE FRACTURE WITH EXTENSION PROXIMALLY INTO FEMORAL SHAFT

    B3. POSTERIOR TANGENTIAL FRACTURE OF ONE OR BOTH CONDYLES

C. BICONDYLAR

    C1. INTERCONDYLAR

    C2. INTERCONDYLAR WITH A COMMINUTED SUPRACONDYLAR COMPONENT

    C3. SEVERLY COMMINUTED BICONDYLAR FRACTURE

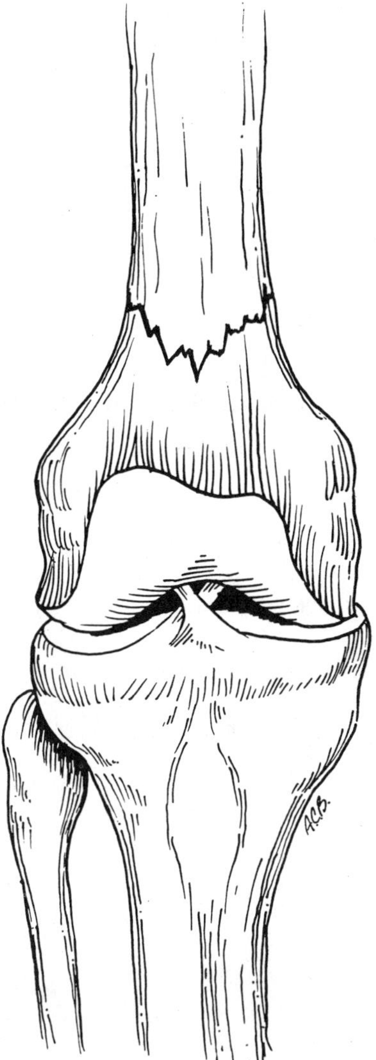
A.C.B.

SUPRACONDYLAR FEMORAL FRACTURES

(AO Classification)

A. EXTRA-ARTICULAR

    A1. AVULSION OF THE MEDIAL OR LATERAL EPICONDYLE

    A2. SIMPLE SUPRACONDYLAR

    A3. COMMINUTED SUPRACONDYLAR

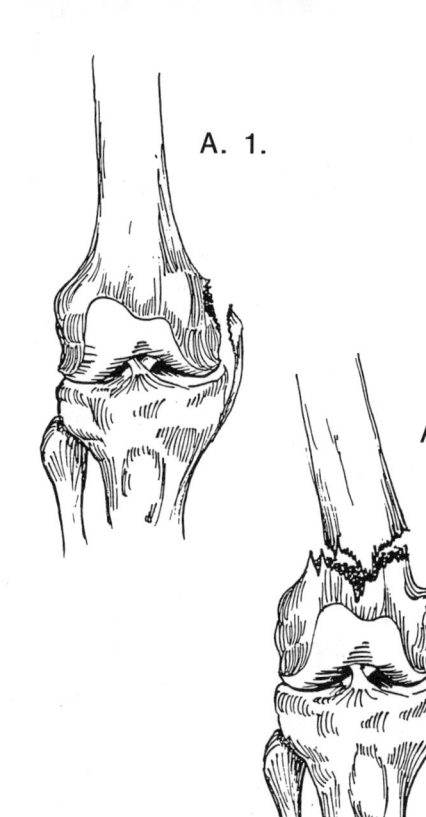

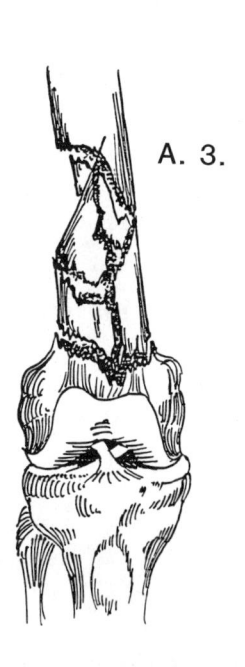

A. 1.

A. 2.

A. 3.

SUPRACONDYLAR FEMORAL FRACTURES

(AO Classification)

B. UNICONDYLAR

    B1. MEDIAL OR LATERAL CONDYLE

    B2. CONDYLE FRACTURE WITH EXTENSION PROXIMALLY INTO FEMORAL SHAFT

    B3. POSTERIOR TANGENTIAL FRACTURE OF ONE OR BOTH CONDYLES

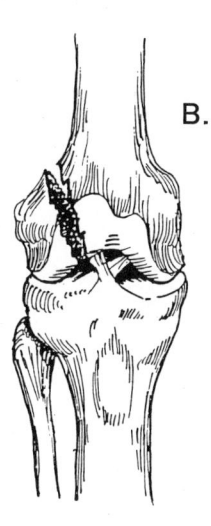

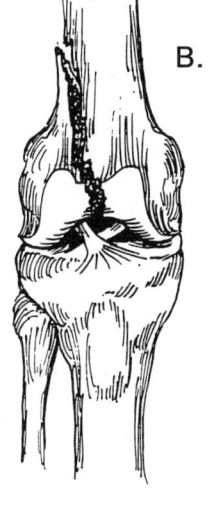

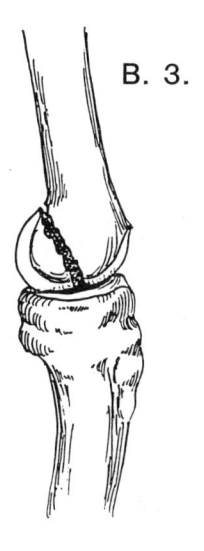

B. 1.

B. 2.

B. 3.

SUPRACONDYLAR FEMORAL FRACTURES

(AO Classification)

C. BICONDYLAR

    C1. INTERCONDYLAR

    C2. INTERCONDYLAR WITH A COMMINUTED SUPRACONDYLAR COMPONENT

    C3. SEVERLY COMMINUTED BICONDYLAR FRACTURE

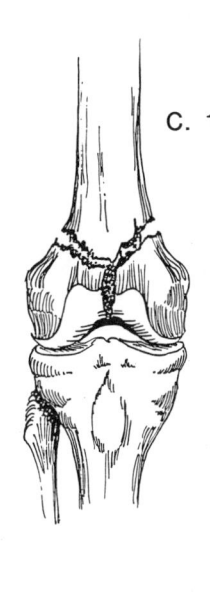

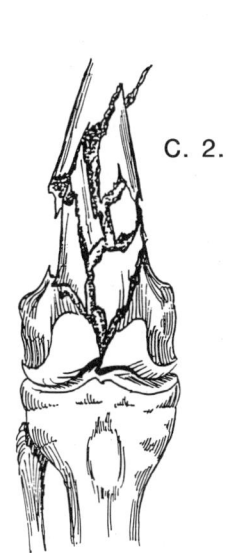

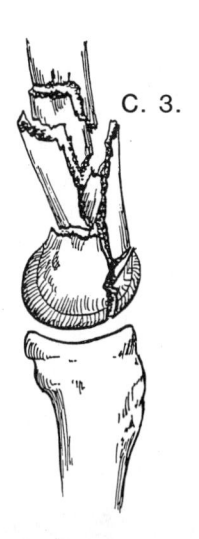

C. 1.

C. 2.

C. 3.

PATELLA FRACTURES

(Fracture Configuration Classification)

I. NONDISPLACED

II. TRANSVERSE

III. UPPER OR LOWER POLE

IV. COMMINUTED

V. VERTICAL

I.

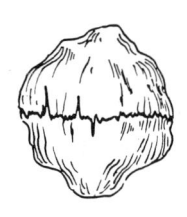

II.

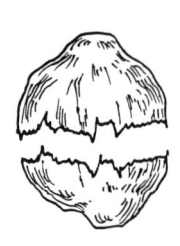

III.

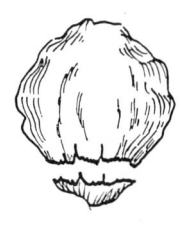

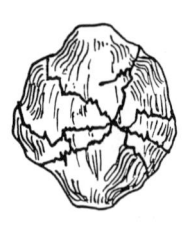

IV.

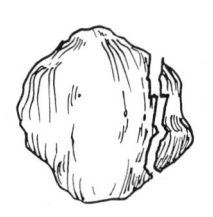

V.

FRACTURES OF THE TIBIAL SPINE

(Meyers Classification)

I. FRACTURE TILTED UP ONLY ANTERIORLY

II. ANTERIOR PORTION LIFTED COMPLETELY FROM TIBIA WITH ONLY SOME POSTERIOR ATTACHMENT

IIIA. INTERCONDYLAR FRAGMENT NOT IN CONTACT WITH THE TIBIA

IIIB. INTERCONDYLAR FRAGMENT ROTATED

I.

II.

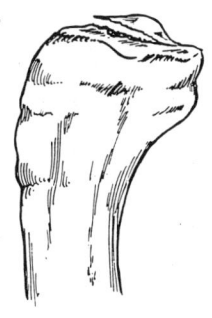

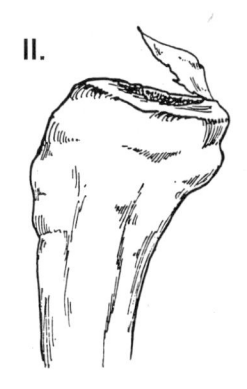

III. A.

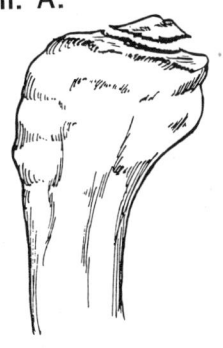

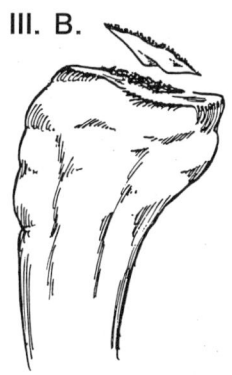

III. B.

FRACTURES OF THE TIBIAL PLATEAU

(Schatzker Classification)

I. CLEAVAGE OR WEDGE TYPE FRACTURES OF THE LATERAL TIBIAL PLATEAU - 24%[a]

II. LATERAL WEDGE FRACTURE WITH ADJACENT DEPRESSION - 26%

III. PURE CENTRAL DEPRESSION WITHOUT AN ASSOCIATED WEDGE FRACTURE - 26%

IV. WEDGE OR DEPRESSION FRACTURES OF THE MEDIAL TIBIAL PLATEAU - 11%

V. BICONDYLAR FRACTURE OF THE TIBIAL PLATEAU - 10%

VI. TIBIAL PLATEAU FRACTURE WITH DISASSOCIATION OF THE METAPHYSIS FROM THE DIAPHYSIS BY A FRACTURE - 3%

[a] *Percentages indicate the frequency of fracture occurrence.*

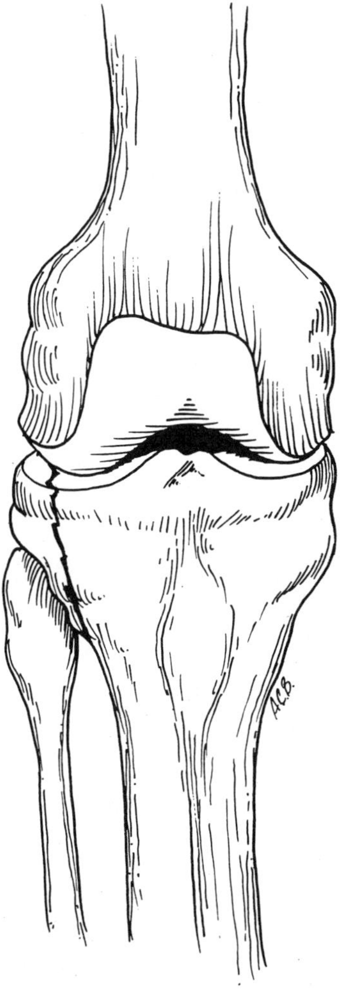
A.C.B.

FRACTURES OF THE TIBIAL PLATEAU

(Schatzker Classification)

I. CLEAVAGE OR WEDGE TYPE FRACTURES OF THE LATERAL TIBIAL PLATEAU

II. LATERAL WEDGE FRACTURE WITH ADJACENT DEPRESSION

III. PURE CENTRAL DEPRESSION WITHOUT AN ASSOCIATED WEDGE FRACTURE

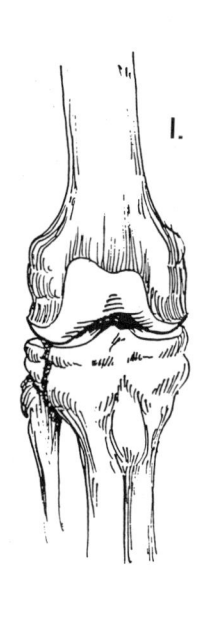

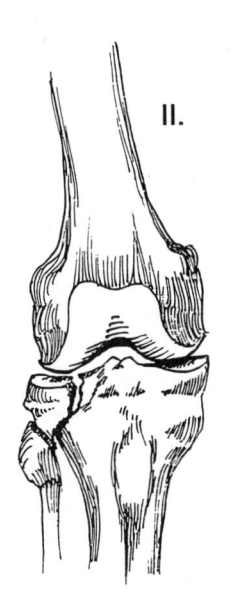

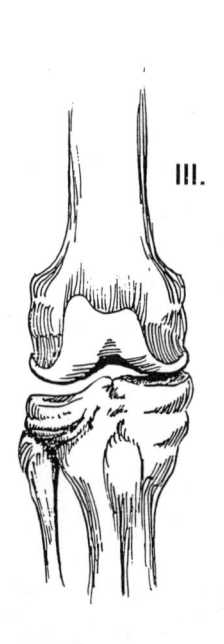

I.

II.

III.

FRACTURES OF THE TIBIAL PLATEAU

(Schatzker Classification)

IV. WEDGE OR DEPRESSION FRACTURES OF THE MEDIAL TIBIAL PLATEAU

V. BICONDYLAR FRACTURE OF THE TIBIAL PLATEAU

VI. TIBIAL PLATEAU FRACTURE WITH DISASSOCIATION OF THE METAPHYSIS FROM THE DIAPHYSIS BY A FRACTURE

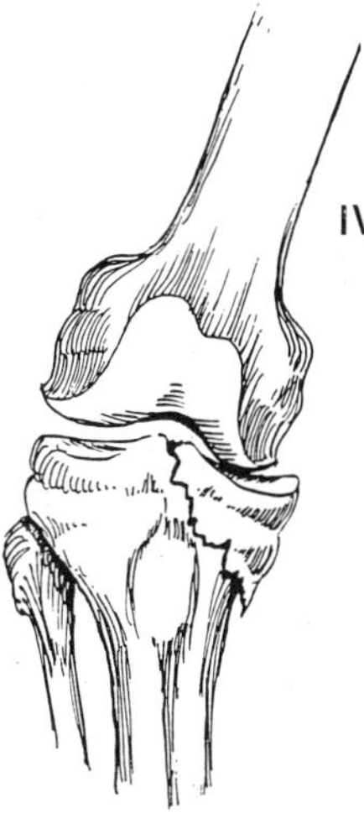

IV.

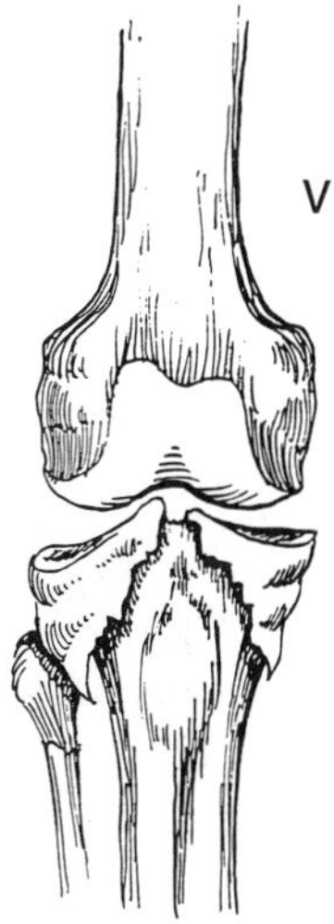

V.

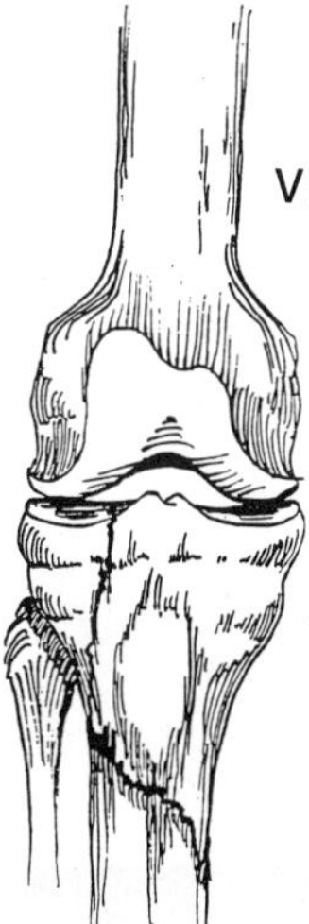

VI.

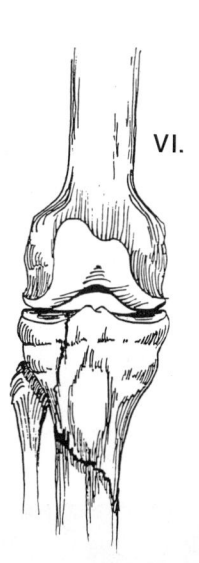

TIBIAL SHAFT FRACTURES

(Chapman Classification)

A. TRANSVERSE OR SHORT OBLIQUE

B. SMALL BUTTERFLY FRAGMENT

C. LARGE BUTTERFLY FRAGMENT

D. SEGMENTAL COMMINUTION

E. SPIRAL

F. PROMIMAL ONE-FOURTH TRANSVERSE OR OBLIQUE

G. DISTAL ONE-FOURTH TRANSVERSE OR OBLIQUE

Type A is usually stable; B and C stability depend on the size of the butterfly fragment.

Type D is usually unstable while types E, F and G are stable but difficult to control.

A.

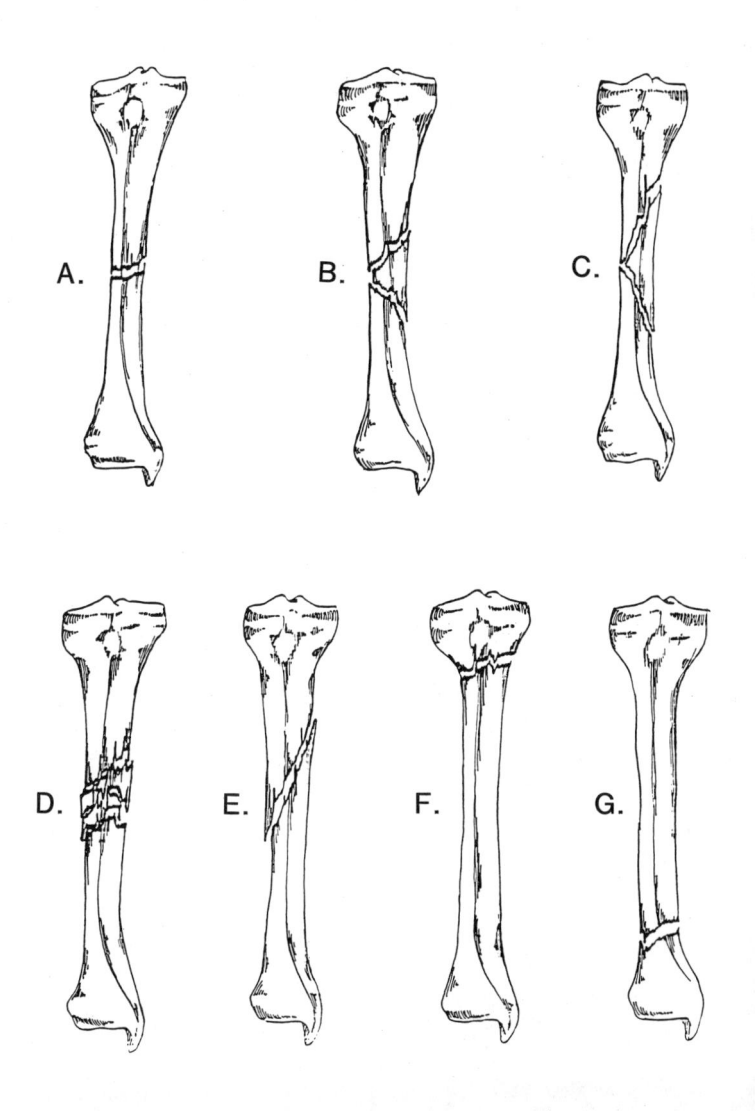

B.

C.

D.

E.

F.

G.

139

FRACTURES OF THE DISTAL TIBIA
WITH INTRA-ARTICULAR EXTENSION - PILON FRACTURE

(AO Classification)

I. CLEAVAGE FRACTURES OF THE ARTICULAR SURFACE WITHOUT SIGNIFICANT DISPLACEMENT

II. CLEAVAGE FRACTURES OF THE ARTICULAR SURFACE WITH SIGNIFICANT ARTICULAR INCONGRUITY, BUT WITHOUT EXTENSIVE COMMINUTION

III. CLEAVAGE FRACTURES OF THE ARTICULAR SURFACE WITH SIGNIFICANT COMPRESSION, DISPLACEMENT, AND COMMINUTION

I.   II.   III.

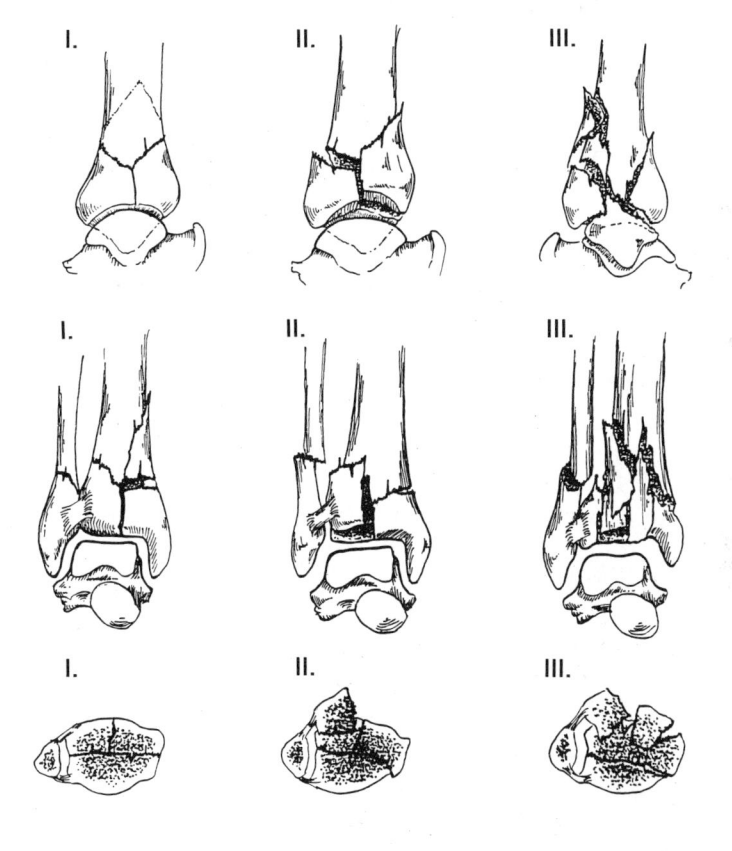

I.   II.   III.

I.   II.   III.

ANKLE FRACTURE CLASSIFICATIONS[a]

(AO Classification)

(Lauge - Hansen Classification)

AO CLASSIFICATION

    A.   TRANSVERSE FIBULA FRACTURE AT OR BELOW JOINT LINE

    B.   SPRAL FIBULA FRACTURE BEGINNING AT JOINT LINE

    C.   OBLIQUE FIBULA FRACTURE ABOVE ANKLE MORTISE

LAUGE - HANSEN CLASSIFICATION

    A.   SUPINATION - EVERSION

    B.   SUPINATION - ADDUCTION

    C.   PRONATION - ABDUCTION

    D.   PRONATION - EVERSION

    E.   PRONATION - DORSIFLEXION

[a] *Two widely used classifications exist for ankle fractures.*

143

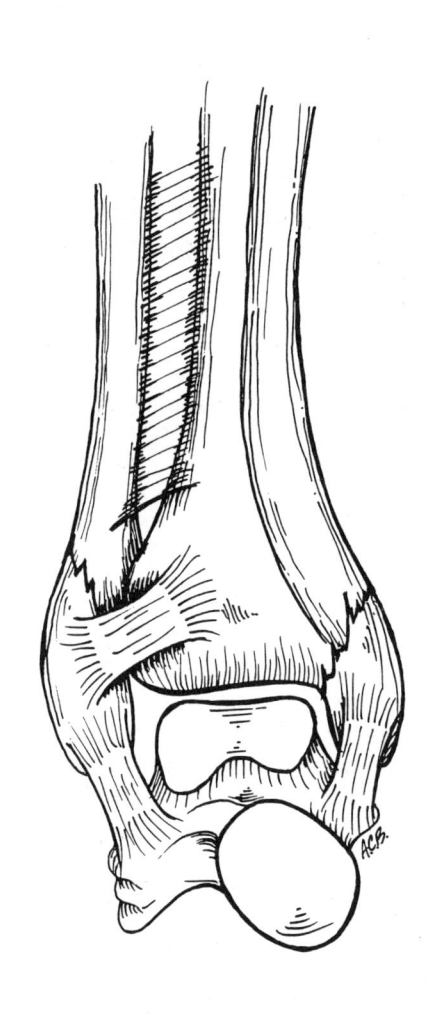

ANKLE FRACTURE CLASSIFICATIONS

(AO Classification)

AO CLASSIFICATION

- A. TRANSVERSE FIBULA FRACTURE AT OR BELOW THE JOINT LINE WITH POSSIBLE SHEAR FRACTURE OF THE MEDIAL MALLEOLUS. TIBIOFIBULAR SYNDESMOSIS INTACT.

- B. SPIRAL FIBULA FRACTURE BEGINNING AT THE JOINT LINE WITH ASSOCIATED MEDIAL INJURY. ANTERIOR SYNDESMOSIS MAY BE TORN BUT POSTERIOR IS USUALLY INTACT. OVERALL INTEGRITY OF THE TIBIOFIBULAR SYNDESMOSIS IS INTACT.

- C1. OBLIQUE FIBULA FRACTURE ABOVE A RUPTURED TIBIOFIBULAR LIGAMENT WITH ASSOCIATED MEDIAL INJURY. TIBIOFIBULAR SYNDESMOSIS IS ALWAYS DISRUPTED.

- C2. OBLIQUE FIBULA FRACTURE WELL ABOVE ANKLE MORTISE WITH EXTENSIVE TIBIOFIBULAR SYNDESMOSIS DISRUPTION.

AO Classification emphasizes the fibula fracture.

The more proximal the fibular fracture, the greater the syndesmosis injury and displacement of the ankle mortise.

A.

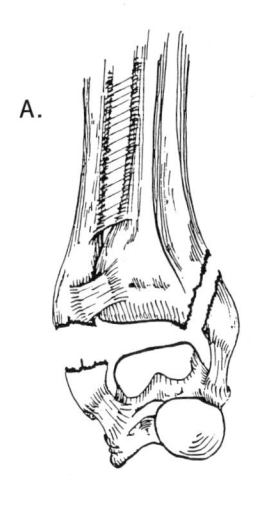

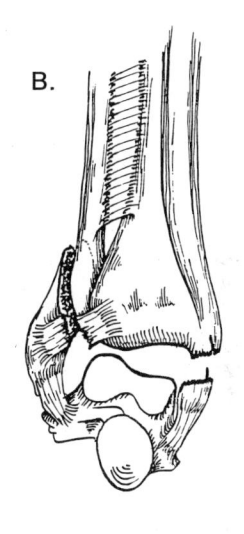

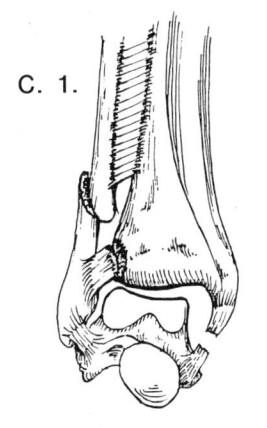

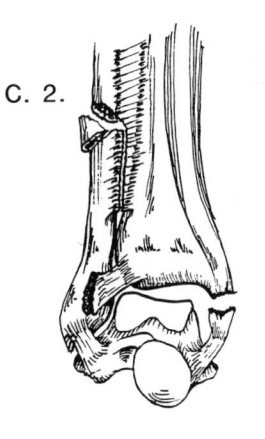

B.

C. 1.

C. 2.

145

ANKLE FRACTURE CLASSIFICATIONS

(Lauge - Hansen Classification)

A. SUPINATION - EVERSION

  I. DISRUPTION OF THE ANTERIOR TIBIOFIBULAR LIGAMENT

  II. SPIRAL OBLIQUE FRACTURE OF THE DISTAL FIBULA

  III. DISRUPTION POSTERIOR TIBIOFIBULAR LIGAMENT, MAY FRACTURE POSTERIOR TIBIA

  IV. MEDIAL MALLEOLUS FRACTURE OR DELTOID LIGAMENT TEAR

B. SUPINATION - ADDUCTION

  I. TRANSVERSE FRACTURE LATERAL MALLEOLUS OR RUPTURE COLLATERAL LIGAMENT

  II. VERTICAL FRACTURE OF MEDIAL MALLEOLUS

SUPINATION - EVERSION is the most common type.

The Lauge - Hansen Classification is based on mechanism of injury. The first word in the classification refers to the position of the foot (SUPINATION or PRONATION) at the time of injury. The second word refers to the direction of the deforming force.

Each of the four injury categories are subdivided into stages indicating increasing severity of injury. Higher stages indicate more severe injury and worse prognosis.

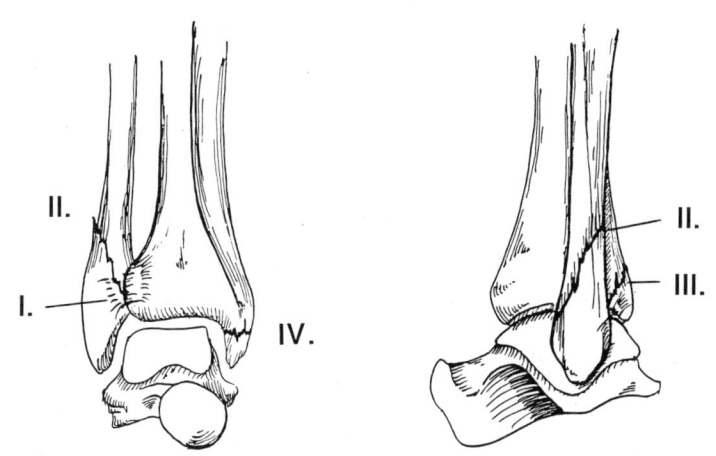

A. Supination Eversion

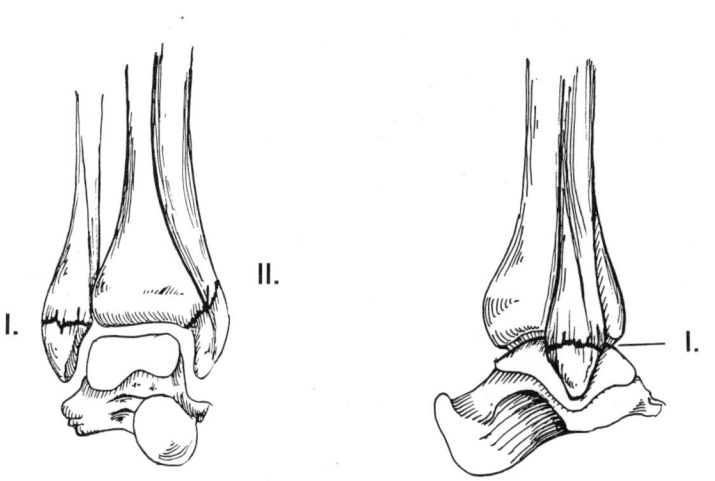

B. Supination Adduction

ANKLE FRACTURE CLASSIFICATIONS

(Lauge - Hansen Classification)

C. PRONATION - ABDUCTION

    I. TRANSVERSE FRACTURE OF THE MEDIAL MALLEOLUS OR DELTOID LIGAMENT RUPTURE

    II. ANTERIOR AND POSTURE TIBIOFIBULAR LIGAMENT RUPTURE WITH OR WITHOUT FRAGMENT OF POSTERIOR MARGIN OF THE TIBIA

    III. SHORT HORIZONTALLY DIRECTED OBLIQUE FIBULA FRACTURE

D. PRONATION - EVERSION

    I. FRACTURE OF THE MEDIAL MALLEOLUS OR RUPTURE OF THE DELTOID LIGAMENT

    II. TEAR OF THE ANTERIOR TIBIOFIBULAR AND INTEROSSEOUS LIGAMENTS

    III. SPIRAL FRACTURE OF THE FIBULA 7 TO 8 CM PROXIMAL TO THE TIP OF THE LATERAL MALLEOLUS

    IV. FRACTURE OF THE POSTERIOR LIP OF THE TIBIA

C. Pronation Adduction

D. Pronation Eversion

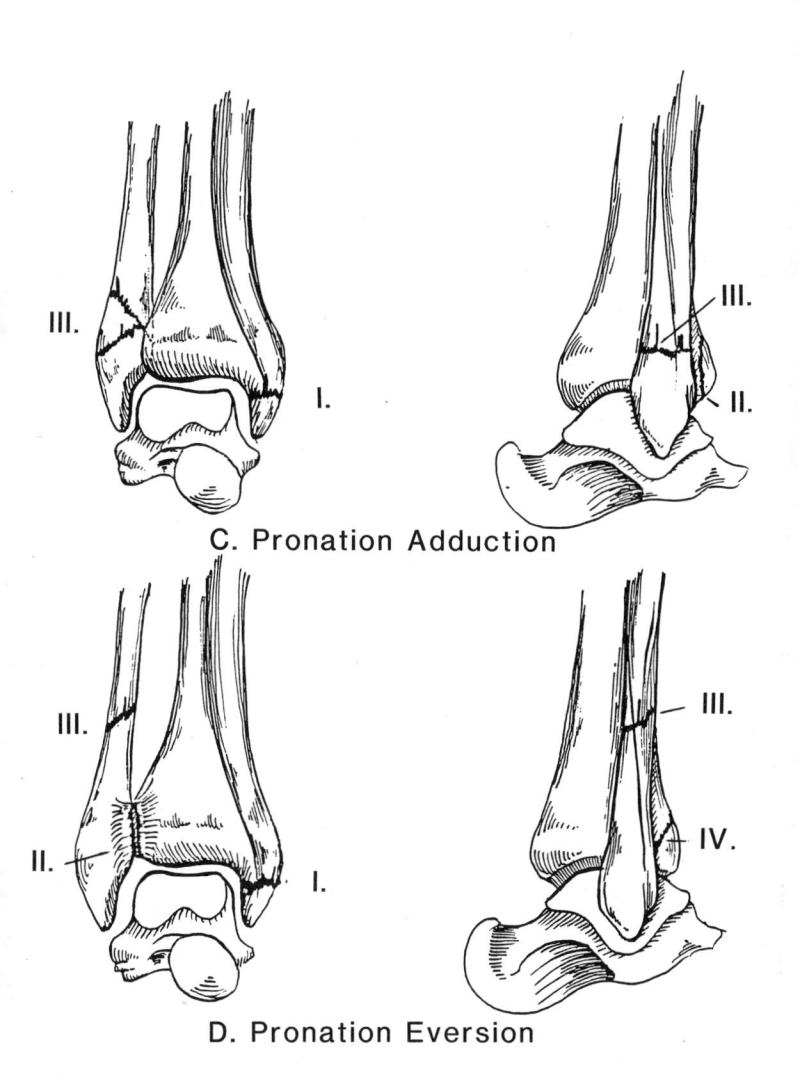

ANKLE FRACTURE CLASSIFICATIONS

(Lauge - Hansen Classification)

E. PRONATION - DORSIFLEXION

    I. FRACTURE OF THE MEDIAL MALLEOLUS OR RUPTURE OF THE DELTOID LIGAMENT

    II. ANTERIOR ARTICULAR TIBIA FRACTURE CAUSED BY DORSIFLEXION OF THE TALUS

    III. SUPRAMALLEOLAR FIBULA FRACTURE

    IV. AVULSION FRACTURE OF THE POSTERIOR TIBIA CAUSED BY CONTINUED DORSIFLEXION OF THE TALUS

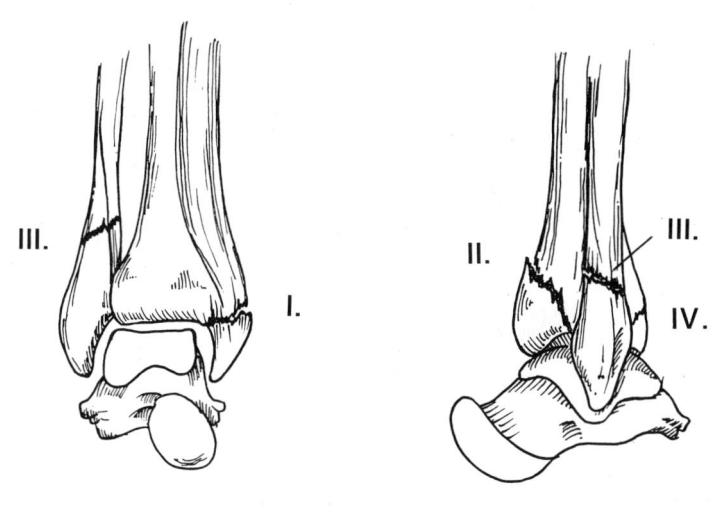

E. Pronation Dorsiflexion

FRACTURES OF THE NECK OF THE TALUS

(Modified Hawkins Classification)

I. NONDISPLACED VERTICAL FRACTURE

II. DISPLACED FRACTURE WITH SUBLUXATION OR DISLOCATION OF THE SUBTALAR JOINT, BUT THE ANKLE MORTISE REMAINS INTACT

III. DISPLACED FRACTURE WITH BOTH SUBTALAR AND TIBIOTALAR DISLOCATIONS

IV. DISPLACED FRACTURE WITH DISLOCATION OF THE NECK FRAGMENT, WHILE THE BODY REMAINS REDUCED

Rate of avascular necrosis of the talus is related to the degree of fracture displacement.

Type IV fractures are rare.

No muscles or tendons originate or insert on talus.

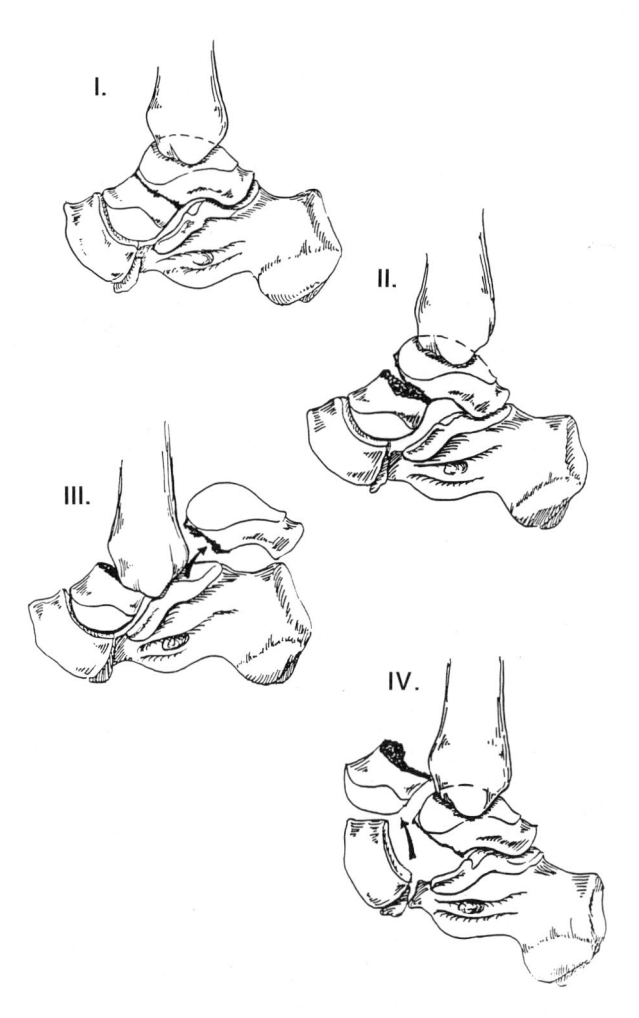

I.

II.

III.

IV.

153

TALAR BODY FRACTURES

(DeLee Classification)

GROUP I. COMPRESSION OR TRANSCHONDRAL FRACTURES OF THE TALAR DOME; INCLUDES OSTEOCHONDRITIS DISSECANS OF THE TALUS

GROUP II. CORONAL, SAGGITAL, OR HORIZONTAL SHEARING FRACTURES OF THE ENTIRE TALAR BODY

GROUP III. POSTERIOR TUBERCLE FRACTURE OF THE TALUS

GROUP IV. LATERAL PROCESS TALAR FRACTURE

GROUP V. TALAR BODY CRUSH FRACTURES

Talar body fractures are uncommon and constitute approximately 1% of all fractures.

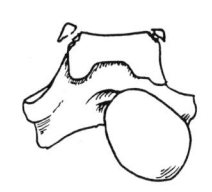

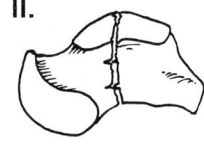

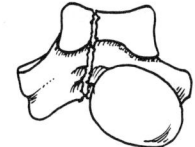

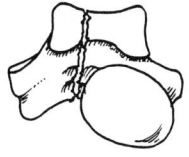

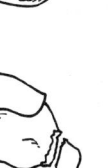

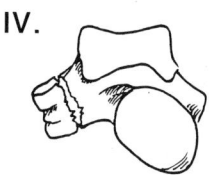

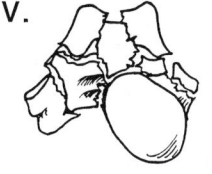

I.

II.

III.

IV.

V.

FRACTURES OF THE CALCANEUS

(Essex - Lopresti Classification)

I. EXTRA-ARTICULAR FRACTURES - 25%[a]

   A. ANTERIOR PROCESS - AVULSION OR COMPRESSION

   B. TUBEROSITY

   C. MEDIAL PROCESS

   D. SUSTENACULUM TALI

   E. BODY WITHOUT INVOLVEMENT OF THE SUBTALAR JOINT

II. INTRA-ARTICULAR FRACTURES - 75%

   A. NONDISPLACED

   B. JOINT DEPRESSION

   C. TONGUE TYPE

   D. SEVERELY COMMINUTED

[a] *Percentages indicate the frequency of fracture occurrence.*

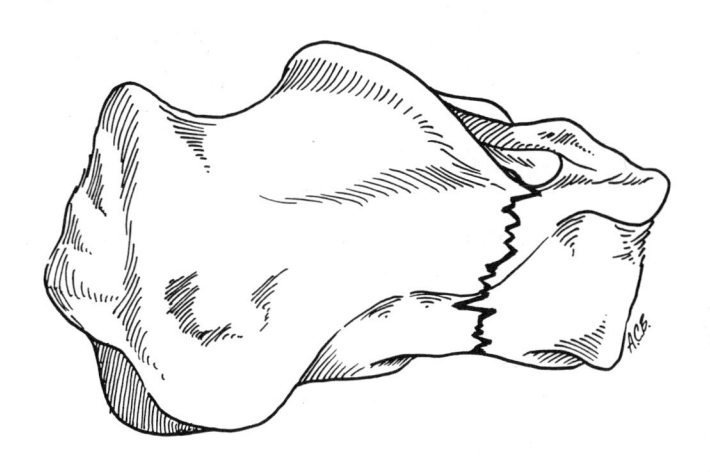

FRACTURES OF THE CALCANEUS

(Essex - Lopresti Classification)

I. EXTRA-ARTICULAR FRACTURES - 25%

    A. ANTERIOR PROCESS - AVULSION OR COMPRESSION

    B. TUBEROSITY

    C. MEDIAL PROCESS

    D. SUSTENACULUM TALI

    E. BODY WITHOUT INVOLVEMENT OF THE SUBTALAR JOINT

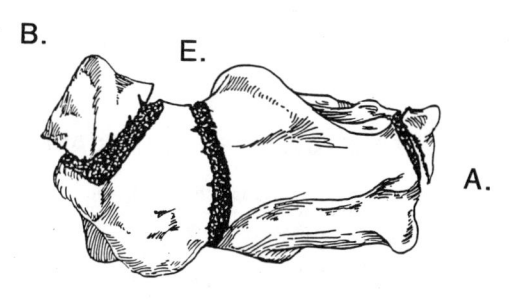

Lateral View

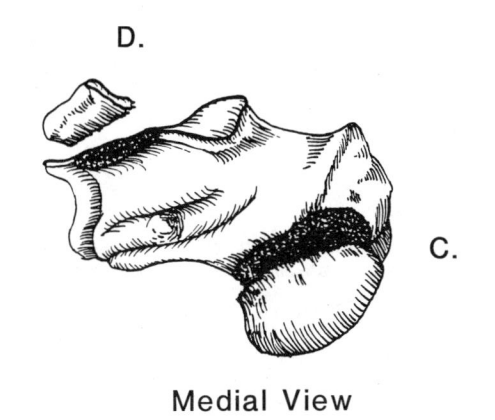

Medial View

FRACTURES OF THE CALCANEUS

(Essex - Lopresti Classification)

II. INTRA-ARTICULAR FRACTURES - 75%

    A. NONDISPLACED

    B. JOINT DEPRESSION

    C. TONGUE TYPE

    D. SEVERELY COMMINUTED

INTRA-ARTICULAR CALCANEUS FRACTURES are frequently associated with other injuries, including ipsilateral lower extremity injuries and thoracolumbar spine fractures.

A.

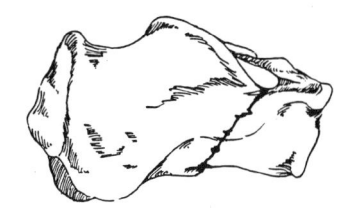

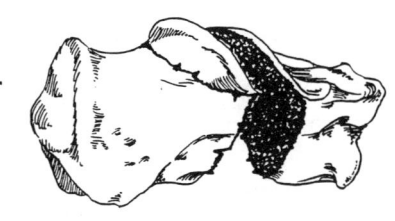

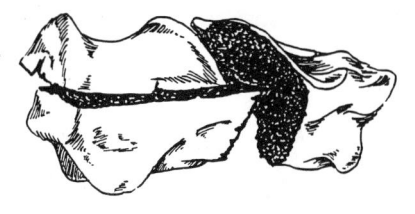

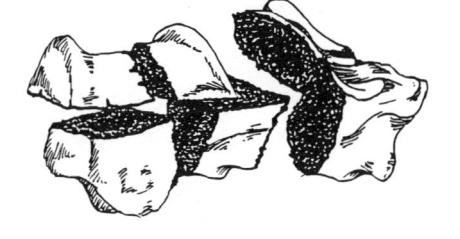

B.

C.

D.

161

CLASSIFICATION OF OPEN FRACTURES

(Gustilo Classification)

I. LOW ENERGY WOUND THAT IS USUALLY LESS THAN 1 CM, OFTEN CAUSED BY BONE PIERCING THE SKIN

II. WOUND GREATER THAN 1 CM IN LENGTH WITH MODERATE AMOUNT OF SOFT TISSUE DAMAGE SECONDARY TO HIGHER ENERGY

III. HIGH ENERGY WOUND THAT IS USUALLY GREATER THAN 1 CM WITH EXTENSIVE SOFT TISSUE DAMAGE

Certain factors always constitute a Type III open fracture: high velocity gunshot wound, shotgun wound, segmental fracture, concommitant major vascular injury, significant diaphyseal bone loss, fracture occurring in a farmyard environment or by the crushing of a fast moving vehicle.

Type III fractures are further subdivided into IIIA (limited periosteal muscle stripping with adequate soft tissue coverage), IIIB (extensive soft tissue and periosteal stripping without adequate local coverage), and IIIC (associated with arterial injury requiring repair).

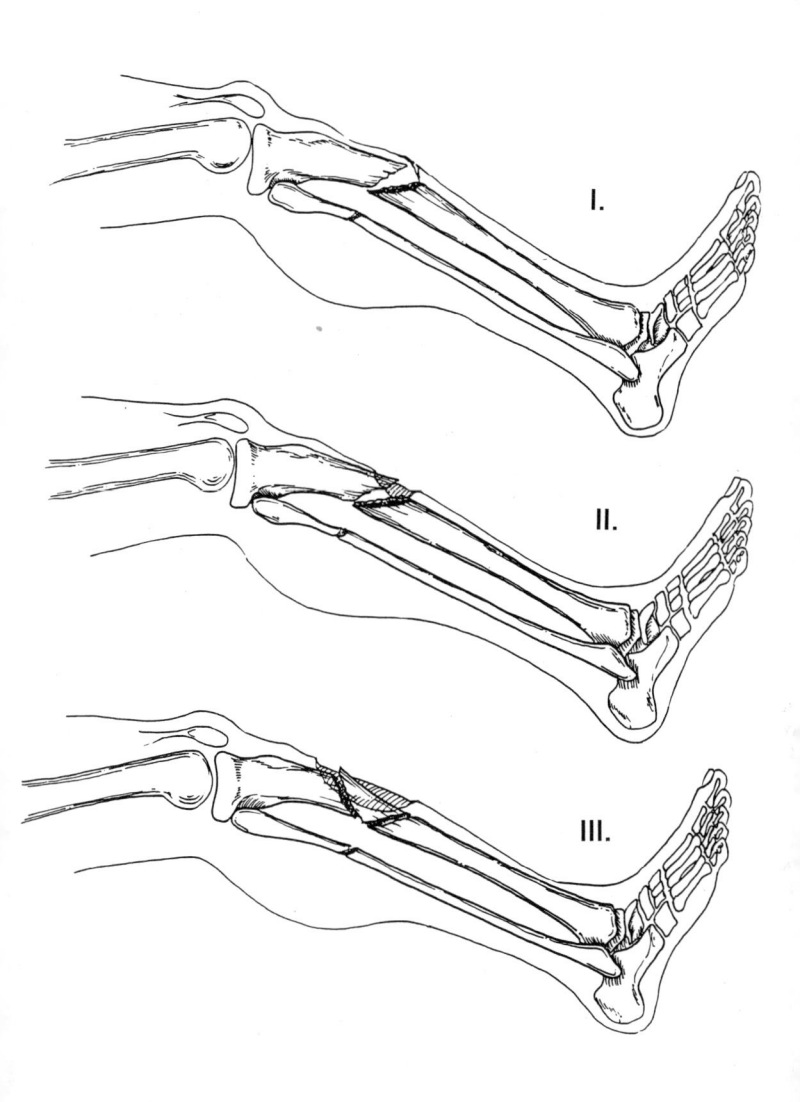

I.

II.

III.

EPONYMS

AVIATOR'S ASTRAGALUS

Implies a variety of fractures of the talus; described after World War I as rudder bar is driven into foot during a plane crash.

BARTON'S FRACTURE

Displaced articular lip fracture of the distal radius; may be associated with carpal subluxation. Fracture configuration may be in a dorsal or volar direction.

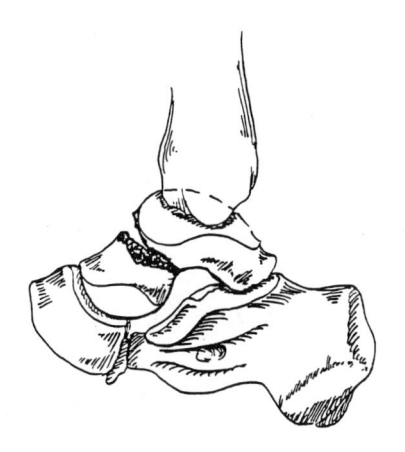

Aviator's Astragalus

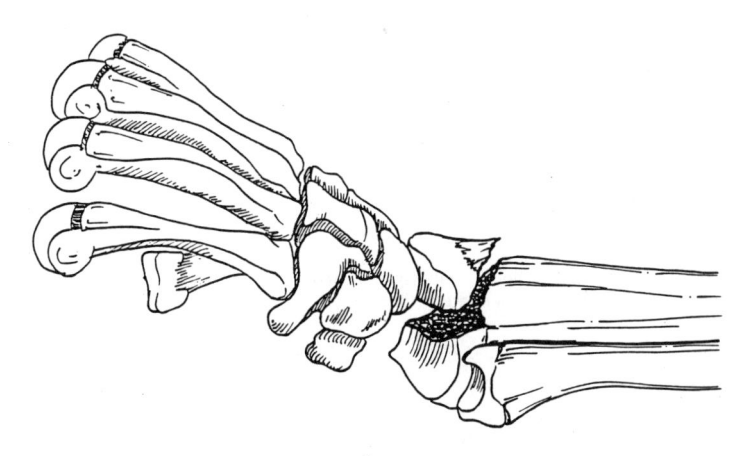

Barton's Fracture

BENNETT'S FRACTURE

Oblique fracture of the first metacarpal base separating a small triangular volar lip fragment from the proximally displaced metacarpal shaft.

BOSWORTH FRACTURE

Fracture of the distal fibula with fixed displacement of the proximal fragment posteriorly behind the posterolateral tibial ridge.

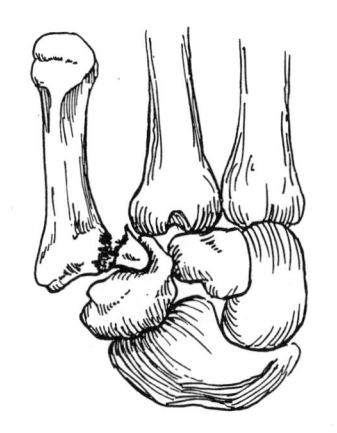

Bennett's Fracture

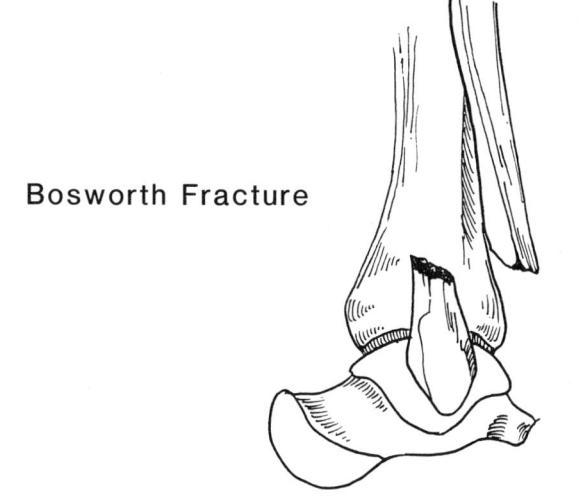

Bosworth Fracture

BOXER'S FRACTURE

Fracture of the fifth metacarpal neck with volar displacement of the metacarpal head.

BURST FRACTURE

Fracture of the vertebral body from axial load, usually with outward displacement of the fragments. May occur in cervical, thoracic, or lumbar spine.

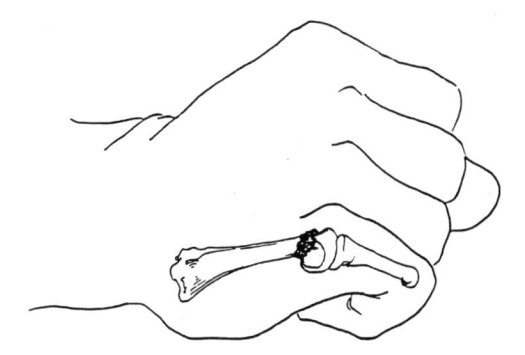

Boxer's Fracture

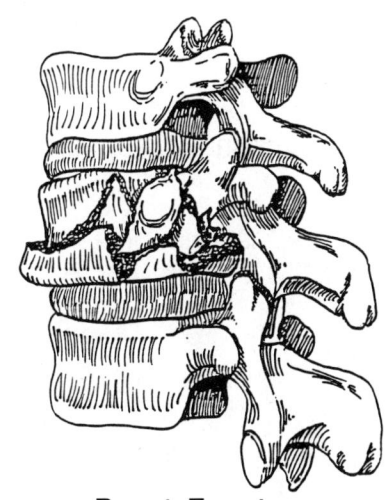

Burst Fracture

CHANCE FRACTURE

Distraction fracture of the thoracolumbar vertebral body with horizontal disruption of the spinous process, neural arch, and vertebral body.

CHAUFFEUR'S FRACTURE (HUTCHINSON'S FRACTURE)

Oblique fracture of the radial styloid, initially attributed to the starting crank of an engine being forcibly reversed by a backfire.

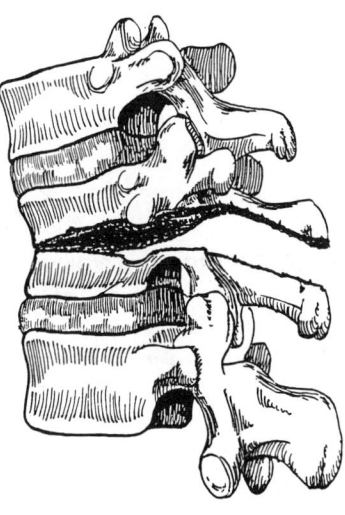

Chance Fracture

Chauffeur's Fracture

(Hutchinson's Fracture)

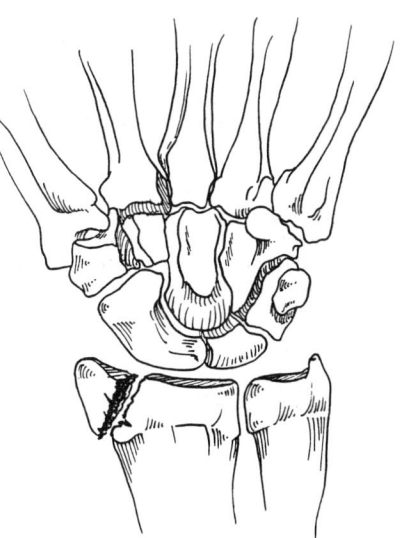

CHOPART'S FRACTURE and DISLOCATION

Fracture and/or dislocation involving Chopart's joints (talonavicular and calcaneocuboid joints) of the foot.

CLAY-SHOVELER'S (COAL-SHOVELER'S) FRACTURE

Spinous process fracture of the lower cervical or upper thoracic vertebrae. Injury initially attributed to workers attempting to throw upwards a full shovel of clay, but the clay adhered to the shovel causing a sudden flexion force opposite to the neck musculature.

Chopart's Fracture

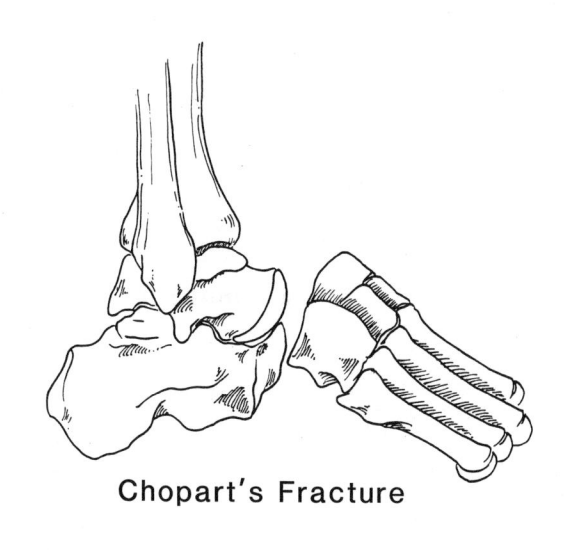

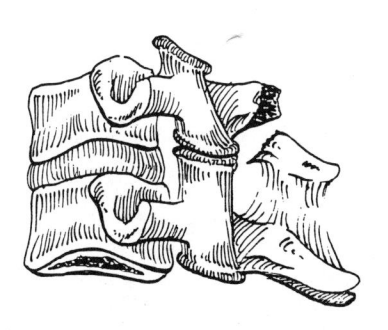

Clay Shoveler's (Coal Shoveler's) Fracture

COLLES' FRACTURE

General term for fractures of the distal radius with dorsal displacement, with or without an ulnar styloid fracture. See Frykman's classification for further details.

COTTON'S FRACTURE

Trimalleolar ankle fracture with fractures of both malleoli and posterior lip of the tibia.

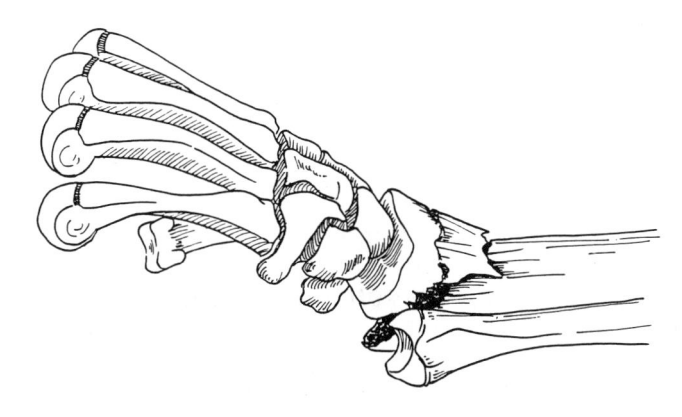

Colle's Fracture

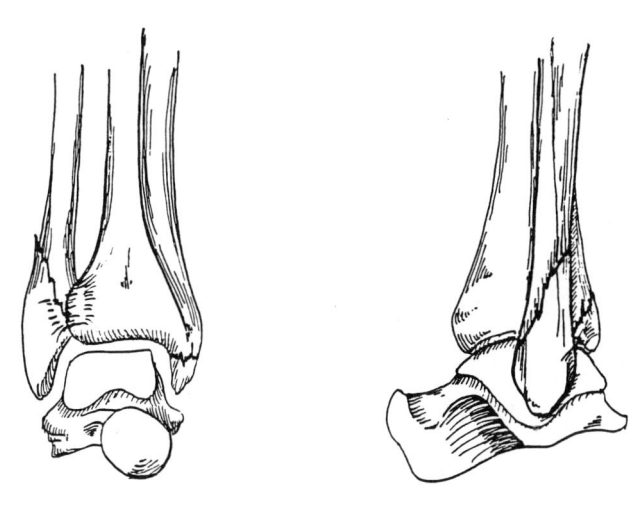

Cotton's Fracture

DIE PUNCH FRACTURE

Intra-articular distal radius fracture with impaction of the dorsal aspect of the lunate fossa.

DUPUYTREN'S FRACTURE

Fracture of the distal fibula with rupture of the distal tibiofibular ligaments and lateral displacement of the talus.

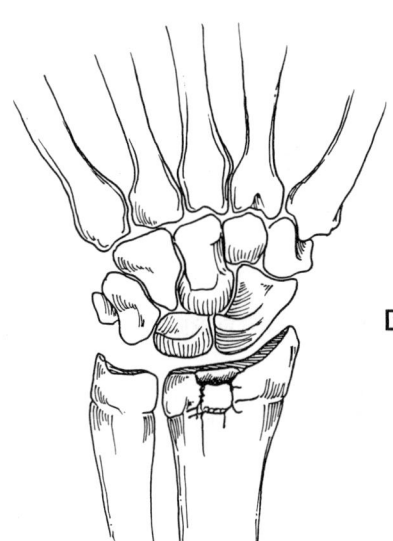

Die Punch Fracture

Dupuytren's Fracture

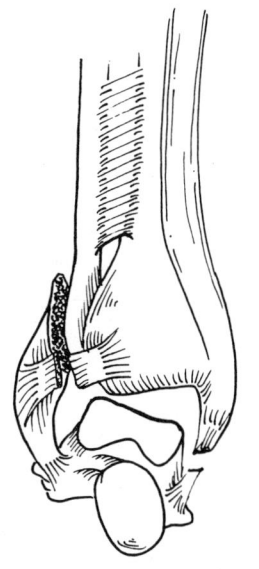

DUVERNEY'S FRACTURE

Fracture of the iliac wing without disruption of the pelvic ring.

ESSEX - LOPRESTI'S FRACTURE

Radial head fracture with associated dislocation of the distal radioulnar joint.

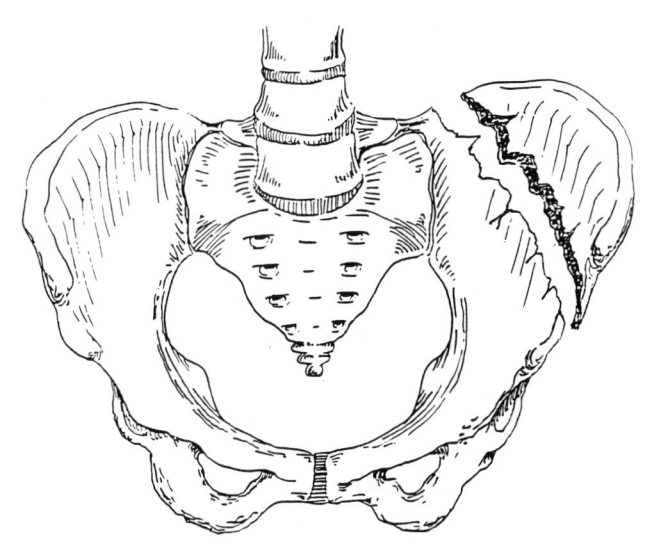

Duverney's Fracture

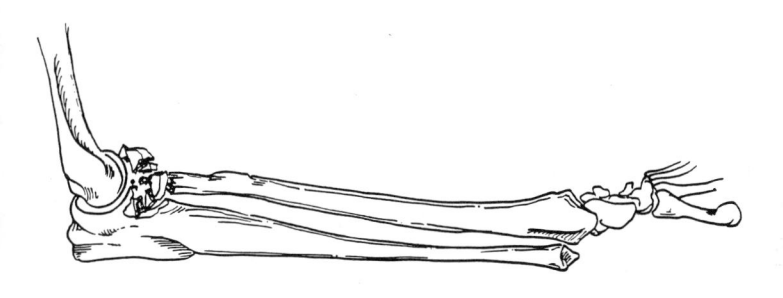

Essex-Lopresti's Fracture

GALEAZZI'S FRACTURE

Fracture of the radius in the distal third associated with subluxation of the distal ulna.

GREENSTICK FRACTURE

Incompletely fractured bone in a child, with a portion of the cortex and periosteum remaining intact on the compression side of the fracture.

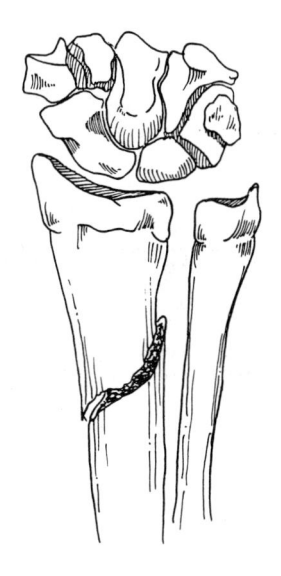

Galeazzi's Fracture

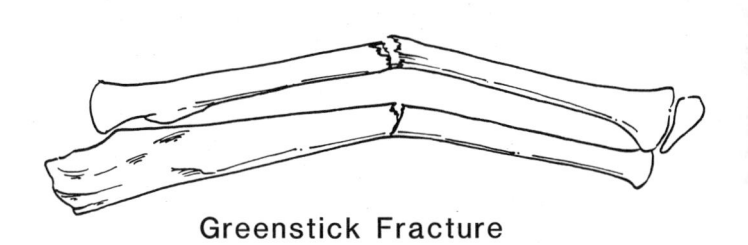

Greenstick Fracture

HAHN - STEINTHAL FRACTURE

Fracture of the capitellum involving a large osseous portion and may involve adjacent trochlea. See classification section for further details of capitellum fractures.

HANGMAN'S FRACTURE

Fracture through the neural arch of the second cervical vertebrae (axis).

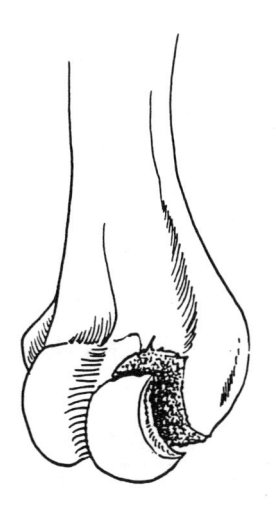

Hahn-Steinthal Fracture

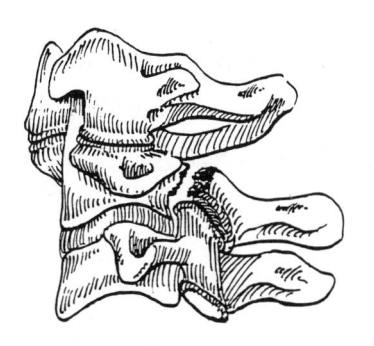

Hangman's Fracture

HILL - SACHS FRACTURE

Posterolateral humeral head compression fracture caused by anterior glenohumeral dislocation and impaction of the humeral head against the anterior glenoid rim.

HOLSTEIN - LEWIS FRACTURE

Fracture of the distal third of the humerus with entrapment of the radial nerve.

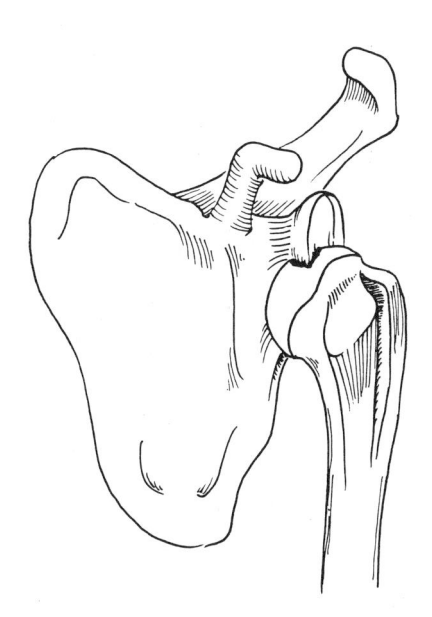

Hill-Sachs
Fracture

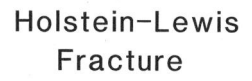

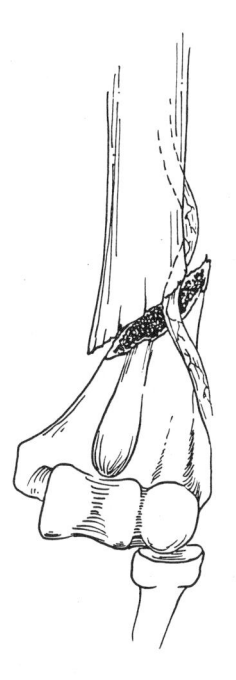

Holstein-Lewis
Fracture

HUTCHINSON'S FRACTURE

See CHAUFFEUR'S FRACTURE, p. 172.

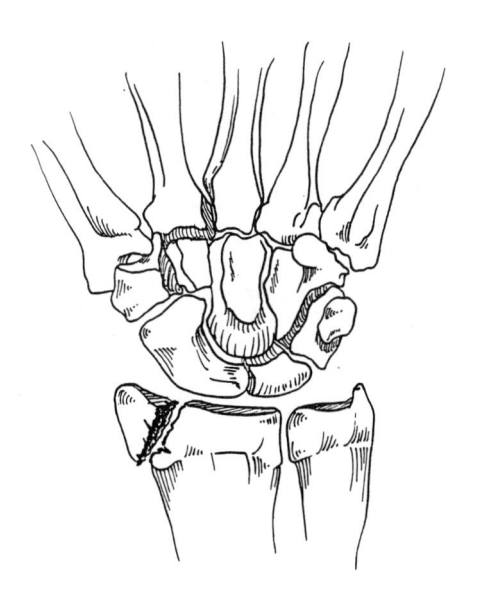

Hutchinson's Fracture

JEFFERSON'S FRACTURE

Comminuted fracture of the ring of the atlas due to axial compressive forces. Fractures usually occur anterior and posterior to the lateral facet joints.

JONES FRACTURE

Diaphyseal fracture of the base of the fifth metatarsal.

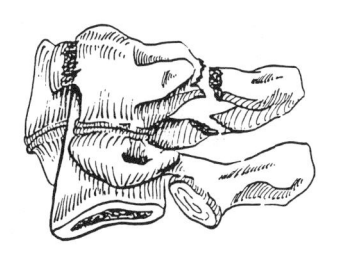

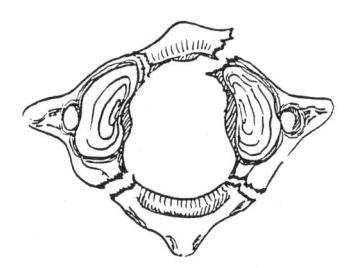

Jefferson's Fracture

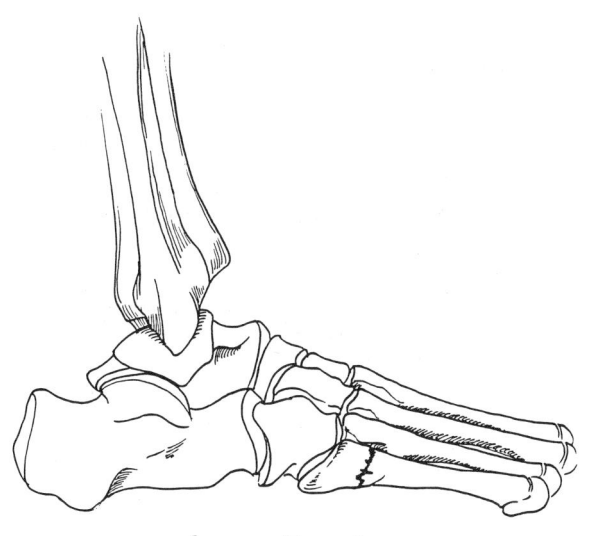

Jones Fracture

KOCHER - LORENZ FRACTURE

Slice fracture of the capitellum involving articular cartilage with minimal subchondral bone. See classification section for further details of capitellum fractures.

LISFRANC'S FRACTURE DISLOCATION

Fracture and/or dislocation involving Lisfranc's (tarsometatarsal) joint of the foot. Lisfranc was one of Napoleon's surgeons and described traumatic foot amputation through the tarsometatarsal joint level.

Kocher-Lorenz
Fracture

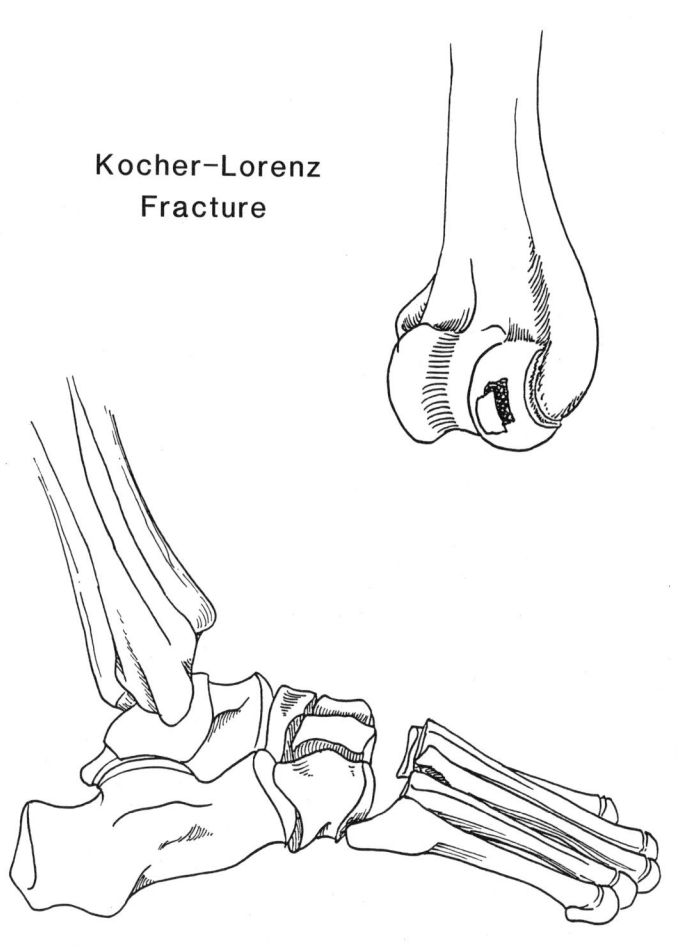

Lisfranc's Fracture Dislocation

MAISONNEUVE'S FRACTURE

Fracture of the proximal fibula with syndesmosis rupture and associated medial malleolus fracture or deltoid ligament rupture.

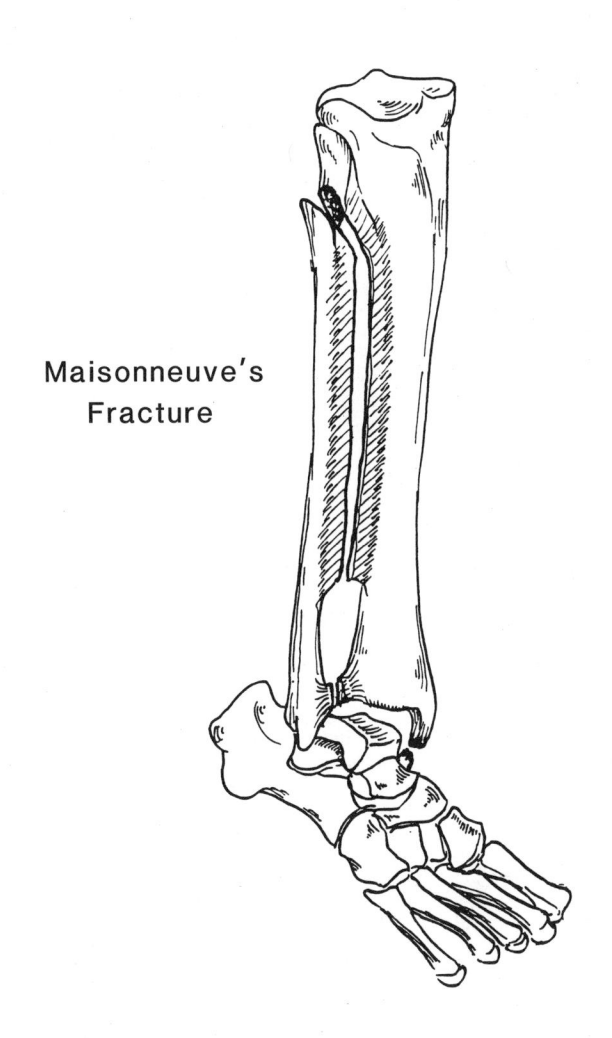

Maisonneuve's Fracture

MALGAIGNE'S FRACTURE

Unstable pelvic fracture with vertical fractures anterior and posterior to the hip joint.

MALLET FINGER

Flexion deformity of the distal interphalangeal joint caused by extensor tendon separation from the distal phalanx. The deformity may be secondary to direct injury of the extensor tendon or an avulsion fracture from the dorsum of the distal phalanx where the tendon inserts.

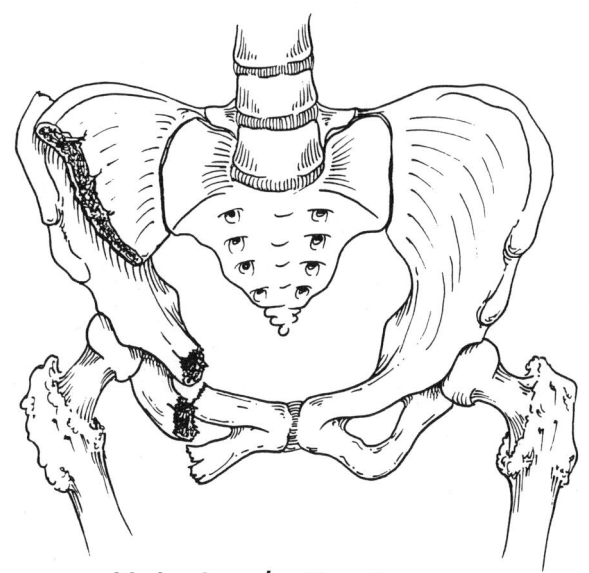

Malgaigne's Fracture

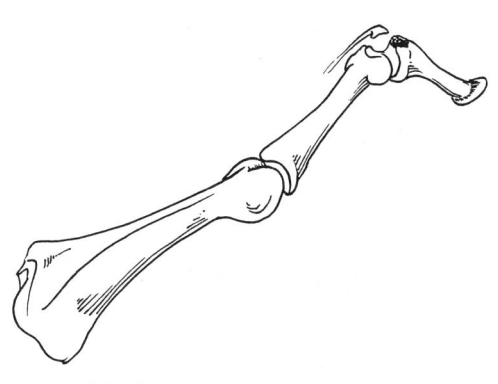

Mallet Finger

MONTEGGIA'S FRACTURE

Fracture of the proximal third of the ulna with associated dislocation of the radial head. Fracture complex has been further classified by Bado; see classification section.

NIGHTSTICK FRACTURE

Isolated fracture of the ulna secondary to direct trauma.

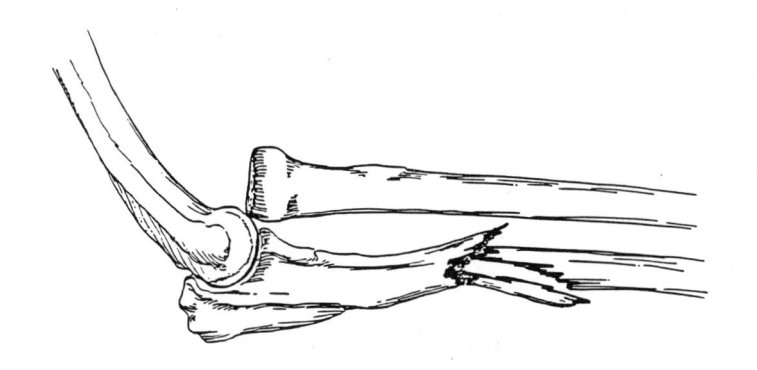

Monteggia's Fracture

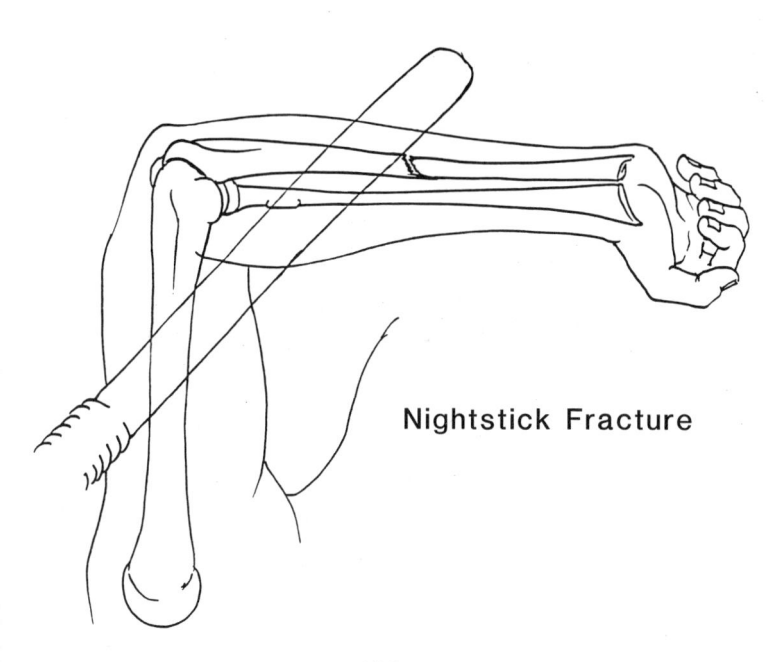

Nightstick Fracture

POSADAS' FRACTURE

Transcondylar humerus fracture with displacement of the distal fragment anteriorly and dislocation of the radius and ulna from the bicondylar fragment.

POTT'S FRACTURE

Fracture of the fibula within 2 to 3 inches above the lateral malleolus with rupture of the deltoid ligament and lateral subluxation of the talus. Pott did not describe disruption of the tibiofibular ligaments.

Posadas' Fracture

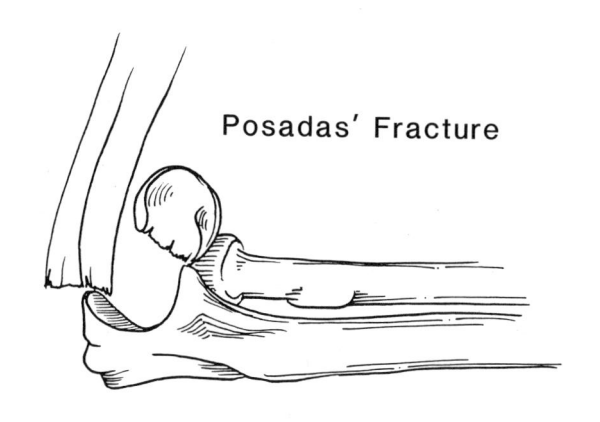

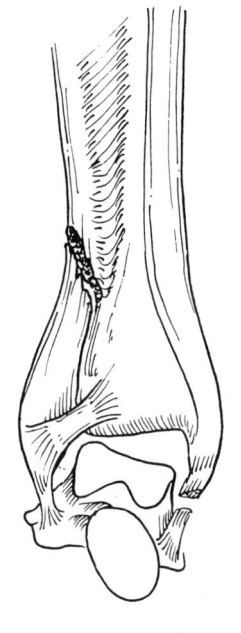

Pott's Fracture

ROLANDO'S FRACTURE

Y-shaped intra-articular fracture of the thumb metacarpal.

SEGOND'S FRACTURE

Avulsion fracture of the lateral tibial condyle from the bony insertion of the iliotibial band.

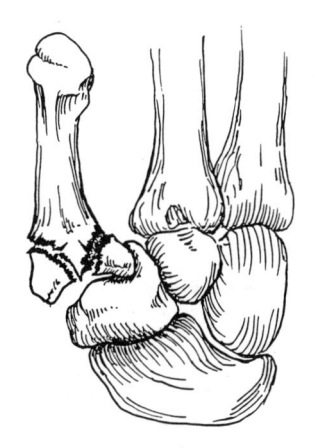

Rolando's Fracture

Segond's Fracture

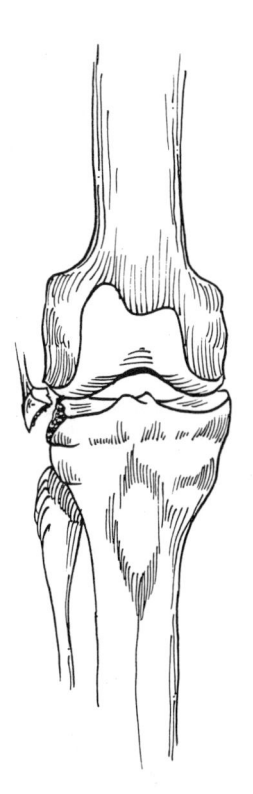

SHEPHERD'S FRACTURE

Fracture of the lateral tubercle of the posterior talar process.

SMITH'S FRACTURE

Fracture of the distal radius with palmar displacement of the distal fragment. Also referred to as a reverse Colles' fracture.

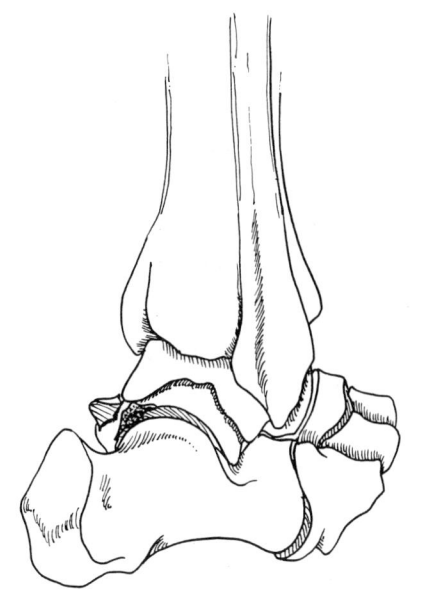

Shepherd's Fracture

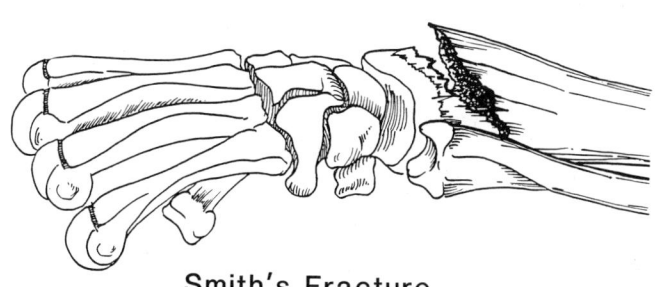

Smith's Fracture

STIEDA'S FRACTURE

Avulsion fracture of the medial femoral condyle at the origin of the medial collateral ligament.

STRADDLE FRACTURE

Bilateral fractures of the superior and inferior pubic rami.

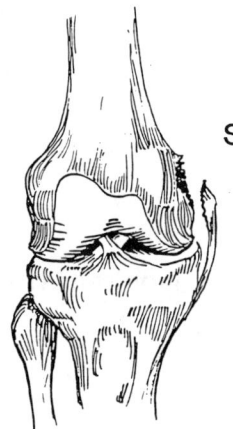

Stieda's Fracture

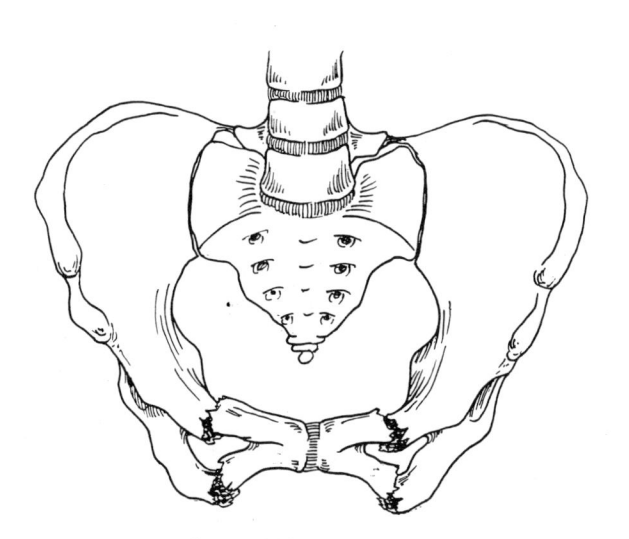

Straddle Fracture

TEARDROP FRACTURE

Flexion fracture dislocation of the cervical spine with associated triangular anterior fragment of the involved vertebrae. Injury complex is unstable with posterior ligamentous disruption.

TILLAUX'S FRACTURE

Fracture of the lateral half of the distal tibial physis during differential closure of the physis. The medial part of the tibial physis has already fused.

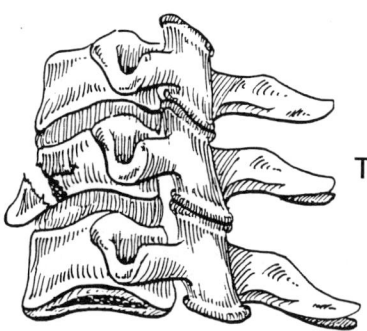

Teardrop Fracture

Tillaux's Fracture

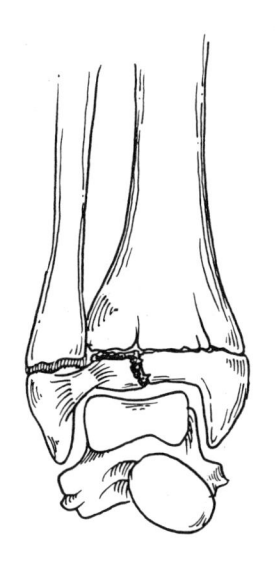

TORUS FRACTURE

Impaction fracture of childhood as the bone buckles instead of fracturing completely.

WALTHER'S FRACTURE

Ischioacetabular fracture which passes through the pubic rami and extends toward the sacroiliac joint. The medial wall of the acetabulum is displaced inward.

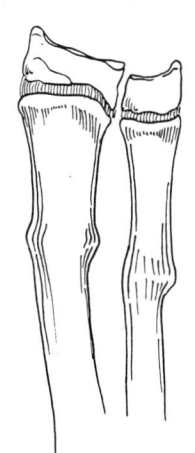

Torus Fracture

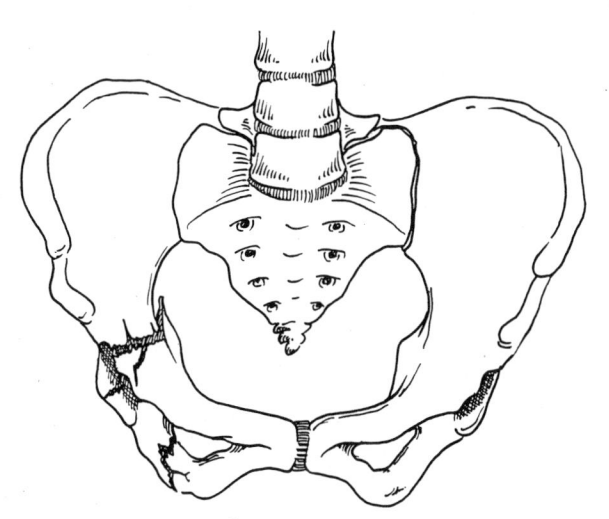

Walther's Fracture

REFERENCES

Anderson, H.G. *The Medical and Surgical Aspects of Aviation.* Oxford University Press, London, 1919.

Anderson, L.D. Fractures of the Shafts of the Radius and Ulna. *In* Rockwood, C.A., and Green, D.P. (Eds.). *Fractures in Adults, Second Edition.* J.B. Lippincott, Philadelphia, 1984, pp. 511-558.

Anderson, L.D, and D'Alonzo, R.T. Fractures of the Odontoid Process of the Axis. *J. Bone Joint Surg.* **46A**: 210-233, 1970.

Ashhurst, A.P.C. An Anatomical and Surgical Study of Fractures of the Lower End of the Humerus. *The Samuel D. Gross Prize Essay of the Philadelphia Academy of Surgery, 1910.* Lea and Febiger, Philadelphia, 1910.

Bado, J.L. The Monteggia Lesion. *Clin. Orthoped.* **50**: 71-86, 1967.

Barton, J.R. Views and Treatment of an Important Injury to the Wrist. *Med. Examiner* **1**: 365, 1838.

Baumann, J.U., and Campbell, R.D., Jr. Significance of Architectural Types of Fractures of the Carpal Scaphoid and Relation to Timing of Treatment. *J. Trauma* **2**: 431-438, 1962.

Bennett, E.H. Fractures of the Metacarpal Bones. *Dublin J. Med. Sci.* **73**: 72-75, 1882.

Bosworth, D.M. Fracture Dislocation of the Ankle with Fixed Displacement of the Fibula Behind the Tibia. *J. Bone Joint Surg.* **29**: 130-135, 1947.

Bryan, R.S. Fractures About the Elbow in Adults. *AAOS Instructional Course Lectures* **30**: 200-223, 1981.

Bryan, R.S., and Morrey, B.F. Fractures of the Distal Humerus. *In* Morrey, B.F. (Ed.). *The Elbow and Its Disorders.* W.B. Saunders, Philadelphia, 1985, pp. 325-327.

Bucholz, R.W., and Gill, K. Classification of Injuries of the Thoracolumbar Spine. *Orthoped. Clin. North. Am.* **17**: 67-73, 1986.

Cancelmo. J.J., Jr. Clay-Shoveler's Fracture. A Helpful Diagnostic Sign. *Am. J. Roentgenol.* **115**: 540, 1972.

Cass, J.R. Fractures and Dislocations Involving the Midfoot. *In* Chapman, M.W. (Ed.). *Operative Orthopaedics.* J.B. Lippincott, Philadelphia, 1988, pp. 1737-1755.

Chance, C.Q. Note on a Type of Flexion Fracture of the Spine. *Br. J. Radiol.* **21**: 452-453, 1948.

Chapman, M.W. (Ed.). *Operative Orthopaedics.* J.B. Lippincott, Philadelphia, 1988.

Chutro, P. *Fractures de la Extremidad Inferior del Humero en los Ninos.* Theses J. Peuser, Buenos Aires, 1904.

Colles, A. On the Fracture of the Carpal Extremity of the Radius. *Edinb. Med. Surg. J.* **10**: 182-186, 1814.

Colton, C.L. Fractures of the Olecranon in Adults: Classification and Management. *Injury* **5**: 121-129, 1973-74.

Cotton, F.J. A New Type of Ankle Fracture. *J. Am. Med. Assoc.* **64**: 318-321, 1915.

DeLee, J.S. Fractures and Dislocations of the Foot. *In* Mann, R.A. (Ed.). *Surgery of the Foot.* C.V. Mosby, St. Louis, 1986, pp. 592-714.

Denis, F. The Three Column Spine and Its Significance in the Classification of Acute Thoracolumbar Spinal Injuries. *Spine* **8**: 817-831, 1983.

Denis, F., Davis, S., and Comfort, T. Sacral Fractures: An Important Problem. *Clin. Orthoped.* **227**: 67-81, 1988.

DePalma, A.F. *The Management of Fractures and Dislocations.* W.B. Saunders, Philadelphia, 1959.

Destot, E. *Injuries of the Wrist.* Ernest Benn, London, 1925.

Dias, L.S. Fractures of the Tibia and Fibula. *In* Rockwood, C.A., and Green, D.P. (Eds.). *Fractures in Children.* J.B. Lippincott, Philadelphia, 1984, pp. 983-1042.

Dimon, J.H., and Hughston, J.S. Unstable Intertrochanteric Fractures of the Hip. *J. Bone Joint Surg.* **49A**: 440-450, 1967.

Dupuytren, G. Of Fractures of the Lower Extremity of the Fibula, and Luxations of the Foot. Reprinted in: *Medical Classics* **4**: 151-172, 1939.

Duverney, J.G. *Traite des Maladies des Os.* Volume 1, DeBure l'Aine', 1751.

Edwards, H.C. Mechanism and Treatment of Backfire Fracture. *J. Bone Joint Surg.* **8**: 701-717, 1926.

Essex-Lopresti, P. Fractures of the Radial Head with Distal Radio-ulnar Dislocation. Report of Two Cases. *J. Bone Joint Surg.* **33B**: 224-247, 1951.

Essex-Lopresti, P. Results of Reduction in Fractures of the Calcaneum. *J. Bone Joint Surg.* **33B**: 284, 1951.

Essex-Lopresti, P. The Mechanism, Reduction Technique, and Results in Fractures of the Os Calcis. *Br. J. Surg.* **39**: 395-419, 1952.

Frykman, G. Fractures of the Distal Radius Including Sequelae - Shoulder, Hand, Finger Syndrome, Disturbance in the Distal Radio-Ulnar Joint and Impairment of Nerve Functions. *Acta. Orthoped. Scand. (Suppl.)* **108**: 1-153, 1967.

Galeazzi, R. Uber ein Besonderes Syndrom bei Verlrtzunger im Bereich der Unter Armknochen. *Arch. Orthop. Unfallchir.* **35**: 557-562, 1934.

Garden, R.S. Stabilty and Union in Subcapital Fractures of the Femur. *J. Bone Joint Surg.* **46B**: 630-647, 1964.

Green, D.P., and O'Brien, E.T. Fractures of the Thumb Metacarpal. *Southern Med. J.* **65**: 807-814, 1972.

Green, D.P., and Rowland, S.A. Fractures and Dislocations in the Hand. *In* Rockwood, C.A., and Green, D.P. (Eds.). *Fractures in Adults, Second Edition.* J.B. Lippincott, Philadelphia, 1984, pp. 313-410.

Gustilo, R.B., and Anderson, J.T. Prevention of Infection in the Treatment of One Thousand and Twenty-Five Open Fractures of Long Bones. Retrospective and Prospective Analyses. *J. Bone Joint Surg.* **58A**: 453-458, 1976.

Gustilo, R.B., Mendoza, R.M., and Williams, D.N. Problems in the Management of Type III (Severe) Open Fractures. A New Classification of Type III Open Fractures. *J. Trauma* **24**: 742-746, 1984.

Hahn, N.F. Fall von eine Besonderes Varietat der Frakturen des Ellenbogens. *Zeitschrift Wundarzte und Geburtshelte* **6**: 185-189, 1853.

Harris, J.H., Edeiken-Monroe, B., and Kopaniky, D.R. A Practical Classification of Acute Cervical Spine Injuries. *Orthoped. Clin. North Am.* **17**: 15-30, 1986.

Hawkins, L.G. Fractures of the Neck of the Talus. *J. Bone Joint Surg.* **47A**: 1170-1175, 1965.

Heckman, J.D. Fractures and Dislocations of the Foot. *In* Rockwood, C.A., and Green, D.P. (Eds.). *Fractures in Adults, Second Edition.* J.B. Lippincott, Philadelphia, 1984, pp. 1703-1832.

Hill, H.A., and Sachs, M.D. The Grooved Defect of the Humeral Head. A Frequently Unrecognized Complication of Dislocations of the Shoulder Joint. *Radiology* **35**: 690-700, 1940.

Holstein, A., and Lewis, G.B. Fractures of the Humerus with Radial Nerve Paralysis. *J. Bone Joint Surg.* **45A**: 1382, 1963.

Holdsworth, F.W. Fractures, Dislocations, and Fracture-dislocations of the Spine. *J. Bone Joint Surg.* **45B**: 6-20, 1963.

Hoppenfield, S., and deBoer, P. *Surgical Exposures in Orthopaedics. The Anatomic Approach.* J.B. Lippincott, Philadelphia, 1984, p. 507.

Ideberg, R. Fractures of the Scapula Involving the Glenoid Fossa. *In* Bateman, J.E., and Welsh, R.P. (Eds.). *Surgery of the Shoulder.* B.C. Becker, New York, 1984, 63-66.

Jefferson, G. Fracture of Atlas Vertebrae: Report of Four Cases, and a Review of Those Previously Recorded. *Br. J. Surg.* **7**: 407-422, 1920.

Johnston, G.W. A Follow-up of One Hundred Cases of Fracture of the Head of the Radius With a Review of the Literature. *Ulster Med. J.* **31**: 51-56, 1962.

Jones, R. Fracture of the Base of the Fifth Metatarsal Bone by Indirect Violence. *Ann. Surg.* **35**: 697-700, 1902.

Kaplan, L. The Treatment of Fractures and Dislocations of the Hand and Fingers. Technic of Unpadded Casts for Carpal, Metacarpal and Phalangeal Fractures. *Surg. Clin. North Amer.* **20**: 1695-1720, 1940.

Kocher, T. *Beitrage zur Kenntniss Einiger Tisch Wichtiger Frakturforman.* Sallman, Basel, 1896, pp. 585-591.

Kyle, R.F., Gustilo, R.B., and Premer, R.F. Analysis of 622 Intertrochanteric Hip Fractures: A Retrospective and Prospective Study. *J. Bone Joint Surg.* **61A**: 216-221, 1979.

Lauge-Hansen, N. Ligamentous Ankle Fractures: Diagnosis and Treatment. *Acta. Chir. Scan.* **97**: 544-550, 1949.

Lorenz, H. Zur Kenntniss der Fraktura Humeri (Eminentiae Capitate). *Deutsche Zeitschr. f. Chir.* **78**: 531-545, 1905.

Maisonneuve, J.G. Recherches sur la Fracture du Perone. *Arch. Gen. Med.* **7**: 165-187, 433-473, 1840.

Malgaigne, J.F. *Treatise on Fractures.* J.B. Lippincott, Philadelphia, 1959.

Mason, J.A., Shutkin, N.M. Immediate Active Motion Treatment of Fractures of the Head and Neck of the Radius. *Surg. Gynecol. Obstet.* **76**: 731-737, 1943.

Meyers, M.H., and McKeever, F.M. Fractures of the Intercondylar Eminence of the Tibia. *J. Bone Joint Surg.* **52A**: 1677-1684, 1970.

Milch, H. Fractures and Fracture Dislocations of the Humeral Condyles. *J. Trauma* **4**: 592-607, 1964.

Monteggia, G.B. *Instituzioni Chirrugiche, Volume 5.* Maspero, Milan, 1814.

Muller, M.E., Allgower, M., Schneider, R., and Willenegger, H. *Manual of Internal Fixation, Second Edition.* Springer-Verlag, New York, 1979.

Neer, C.S., II. Displaced Proximal Humeral Fractures: I. Classification and Evaluations. *J. Bone Joint Surg.* **52A**: 1077-1089, 1970.

Neer, C.S., II. Fractures of the Distal Third of the Clavicle. *Clin. Orthoped.* **58**: 43-50, 1968.

Ogden, J.A. The Uniqueness of Growing Bones. *In* Rockwood, C.A., Wilkens, K.E., and King, R.E. (Eds.). *Fractures in Children.* J.B. Lippincott, Philadelphia, 1984, pp. 1-86.

Pantazopoulus, T., Galanos, P., Voyanas, E., *et al.* Fractures of the Neck of the Talus. *Acta. Orthoped. Scand.* **45**: 296-306, 1974.

Pott, P. *Some Few General Remarks on Fractures and Dislocations.* Hawes, Clarke, Collins; London, 1768.

Regan, W., and Morrey, B. Fractures of the Coronoid Process of the Ulna. *J. Bone Joint Surg.* **71A**: 1348-1354, 1989.

Riseborough, E.J., and Radin, E.L. Intercondylar T Fractures of the Humerus in the Adult. *J. Bone Joint Surg.* **51A**: 130-141, 1969.

Roberts, J.B., and Kelly, J.A. *Treatise on Fractures, Second Edition.* J.B. Lippincott, Philadelphia, 1921.

Rockwood, C.A., Jr., and Green, D.P. (Eds.). *Fractures in Adults, Second Edition.* J.B. Lippincott, Philadelphia, 1984.

Rolando, S. Fracture de la Base du Premier Metcarpien: Et Principalement sur une Variete non Encore Decrite. *Presse Med.* **33**: 303, 1910.

Ruedi, T., and Allgower, M. Fractures of the Lower End of the Tibia into the Ankle Joint. *Injury* **1**: 92, 1969.

Russe, O. Fracture of the Carpal Navicular: Diagnosis, Non-operative Treatment, and Operative Treatment. *J. Bone Joint Surg.* **42A**: 759-768, 1960.

Schatzker, J. Compression in the Surgical Treatment of Fractures of the Tibia. *Clin. Orthoped.* **105**: 220-239, 1974.

Scheck, M. Long Term Follow Up of Treatment of Comminuted Fractures of the Distal End of the Radius by Transfixion with Kirschner Wires and Cast. *J. Bone Joint Surg.* **44A**: 337-351, 1962.

Schneider, R.C., and Kahn, E.A. Chronic Neurological Sequelae of Acute Trauma to the Spine and Spinal Cord. Part I. The Significance of the Acute Flexion or "Teardrop" Fracture-dislocation of the Cervical Spine. *J. Bone Joint Surg.* **38A**: 985-997, 1956.

Segond, P. Rechershes Cliniques et Experimentaelis sur les Epanchements Sanquins du Genou par Entorse. *Prog. Met. (Paris)* **7**: 297, 1879.

Seinsheimer, F. Subtrochantenic Fractures of the Femur. *J. Bone Joint Surg.* **60A**: 300-306, 1978.

Shepherd, F.J. A Hitherto Undescribed Fracture of the Astragalus. *J. Anat. Physiol.* **18**: 79-81, 1882.

Smith, R.W. *A Treatise on Fractures in the Vicinity of Joints, and on Certain Forms of Accidental and Congenital Dislocation.* Hodges and Smith, Dublin, 1854.

Stark, H.H., Bayes, J.H., and Wilson, J.N. Mallet Finger. *J. Bone Joint Surg.* **44A**: 1061-1068, 1962.

Steinthal, D. Die Isolierte Fraktur der Eminentia Capitat in Ellenbogengelenk. *Centrallbl. f. Chirugi* **15**: 17-20, 1898.

Stieda, A. *Arch. f. Klin. Chir.* **85**: 815, 1908.

Tile, M. Pelvic Ring Fractures: Should They be Fixed? *J. Bone Joint Surg.* **70B**: 1-12, 1988.

Tile, M. *Fractures of the Pelvis and Acetabulum.* Williams and Wilkins, Baltimore, 1984.

Walther, C. Recherches Experimentelles sur Certains Fracturas de la Cavietecotyloide. *Bull. Soc. Anat. Paris* **5**: 561, 1891.

Watson-Jones, R. *Fractures and Joint Injuries, Volume 2, 3rd Edition.* Williams and Wilkins, Baltimore, 1946.

Winquist, R.A., Hansen, S.T., Jr., and Clawson, D.K. Closed Intramedullary Nailing of Femoral Fractures: A Report of Five Hundred and Twenty Cases. *J. Bone Joint Surg.* **66A**: 529-539, 1984.

Wood-Jones, F. The Examination of Bodies of 100 Men Executed in Nubia in Roman Times. *Br. Med. J.* **1**: 736-737, 1908.

Wood-Jones, F. The Ideal Lesion Produced by Judicial Hanging. *Lancet* **1**: 53, 1913.

INDEX

A

Acetabulum Fractures: 94 - 101
  Displaced: 94, 96 - 101
  Undisplaced: 94
Anderson Classification: 72 - 73
AO Classification: 120 - 127, 140 - 141, 143 - 145
Ankle Fractures: 142 - 151
Ashurst Classification: 36 - 37
Aviator's Astragalus: 166 - 167

B

Bado Classification: 20 - 21
Barton's Fracture: 166 - 167
Bennett's Fracture: 6, 8 - 9, 168 - 169
Bosworth Fracture: 168 - 169
Boxer's Fracture: 170 - 171
Bryan Classification: 32 - 33
Burst Fracture: 170 - 171

C

Calcaneus Fractures: 156 - 161
Capitellum Fractures: 32 - 33
Cervical Spine Injuries: 60 - 71
  Atlanta-Occipital Disassociation: 60, 70 - 71
  Extension-Rotation: 60, 64 - 65
  Flexion: 60, 62 - 63
  Flexion-Rotation: 60, 64 - 65
  Hyperextension: 60, 68 - 69
  Lateral Flexion: 60, 70 - 71
  Odontoid Fractures: 60, 70 - 71
  Vertical Compression: 60, 66 - 67
Chance Fracture: 172 - 173
Chapman Classification: 138 - 139
Chauffeur's Fracture: 172 - 173
Chopart's Fracture and Dislocation: 174 - 175
Clavicle Fractures: 48 - 51
  Distal: 50 - 51

Clay-Shoveler Fracture: 60, 62 - 63, 174 - 175
Coal-Shoveler Fracture: 60, 62 - 63, 174 - 175
Colles' Fracture: 176 - 177
Colton Classification: 22 - 23
Coronoid Fractures: 24 - 25
Cotton's Fracture: 176 - 177

D

D'Alonzo Classification: 72 - 73
DeLee Classification: 154 - 155
Denis Classification: 74 - 81, 102 - 103
Die Puch Fracture: 178 - 179
Dupuytren's Fracture: 178 - 179
Duverney's Fracture: 180 - 181

E

Elbow Dislocation: 26 - 27
Epiphyseal Fracture: 6, 10 - 11
Essex-Lopresti Classification: 156 - 161
Essex-Lopresti's Fracture: 180 - 181

F

Femoral Fractures: 106, 108 - 127
  Femoral Neck: 106 - 109
  Femoral Shaft: 118 - 119
  Intertrochanteric: 106, 110 - 111
  Subtrochanteric: 106, 112 - 117
  Supracondylar: 120 - 127
Frykman Classification: 14 - 19

G

Galeazzi's Fracture: 182 - 183
Garden Classification: 106 - 109
Glenoid Fractures: 54 - 57
Green Classification: 6 - 11
Greenstick Fracture: 182 - 183

Gustilo Classification: 162 - 163

H

Hahn-Steinthal Fracture: 184 - 185
Hangman's Fracture: 60, 68 - 69, 184 - 185
Harris Classification: 60 - 71
Hawkins Classification, Modified: 152 - 153
Hill-Sachs Fracture: 186 - 187
Hip Fractures: 106 - 111
   Capsule Displacement: 108 - 109
Holstein-Lewis Fracture: 186 - 187
Humeral Fractures: 28 - 47
   Capitellum: 32 - 33
   Distal: 28 - 29
   Humeral Condyles: 30 - 31
   Humeral Intercondylar: 34 - 35
   Humeral Supracondylar: 38 - 39
   Humeral Transcondylar: 36 - 37
   Proximal: 40 - 47
Hutchinson's Fracture: 172 - 173, 188 - 189

I

Ideberg Classification: 54 - 57

J

Jefferson Burst Fracture of Atlas: 60, 66 - 67
Jefferson's Fracture: 190 - 191
Jones Fracture: 190 - 191

K

Kaplan Classification: 4 - 5
Kocher Classification, Modified: 38 - 39
Kocher-Lorenz Fracture: 192 - 193
Kyle Classification: 106 - 107, 110 - 111

L

Lauge-Hansen Classification: 142 - 143, 146 - 151
Lisfranc's Fracture Dislocation: 192 - 193

M

Maisonneuve's Fracture: 194 - 195
Malgaigne's Fracture: 196 - 197
Mallet Finger: 196 - 197
Mason Classification with Johnston Modifications: 26 - 27
Metacarpal Fractures, Base of Thumb: 6 - 11
Meyers Classification: 130 - 131
Milch Classification: 30 - 31
Monteggia Lesion: 20 - 21, 198 - 199
Monteggia's Fracture: 20 - 21, 198 - 199
Morrey Classification: 24 - 25, 32 - 33
Muller Classification: 28 - 29

N

Neer Classification: 40 - 47, 50 - 51
Nightstick Fracture: 198 - 199

O

Odontoid Process Fractures: 72 - 73
Olecranon Fractures: 22 - 23
Open Fractures: 162 - 163

P

Patella Fractures: 128 - 129
Pelvic Disruptions: 84 - 93
   Rotationally and Vertically Unstable: 84, 92 - 93
   Stable: 84, 86 - 87
   Rotationally Unstable and Vertically Stable: 84, 88 - 91
Phalanx Fractures, Distal: 4 - 5
Pilon Fracture: 140 - 141

Posadas' Fracture: 200 - 201
Pott's Fracture: 200 - 201

R

Radin Classification: 34 - 35
Radius Dislocation: 20 - 21
Radius Fractures: 14 - 19, 26 - 27
    Radial Head: 26 - 27
    Distal Radius: 14 - 19
        Extra-Articular: 14, 16 - 17
        Intra-Articular: 14, 16 - 19
    Radiocarpal Joint: 14, 16 - 19
    Radioulnar Joint: 14, 18 - 19
Riseborough Classification: 34 - 35
Rolando's Fracture: 6, 8 - 9, 202 - 203
Russe Classification: 12 - 13

S

Sacral Fractures: 102 - 103
Scaphoid Fractures: 12 - 13
Scapula Fractures: 52 - 57
    Glenoid Fractures: 54 - 57
Schatzker Classification: 132 - 137
Segond's Fracture: 202 - 203
Seinsheimer Classification: 106 - 107, 112 - 117
Shepherd's Fracture: 204 - 205
Smith's Fracture: 204 - 205
Stieda's Fracture: 206 - 207
Straddle Fracture: 206 - 207

T

Talus Fractures: 152 - 155
    Talar Body: 154 - 155
    Talar Neck: 152 - 153
Teardrop Fracture: 208 - 209
Thoracolumbar Spinal Injuries: 74 - 81
    Major Spinal Injuries: 74, 78 - 81
    Minor Spinal Injuries: 74, 76 - 77
Tibial Fractures: 130 - 141, 146 - 149
    Distal Tibia: 140 - 141
    Posterior Tibia: 146 - 149
    Tibial Spine: 130 - 131

    Tibial Plateau: 132 - 137
    Tibial Shaft: 138 - 139
Tile Classification: 84 - 101
Tillaux's Fracture: 208 - 209
Torus Fracture: 210 - 211

U

Ulnar Fractures: 14, 18 - 21
    Distal Ulna: 14, 18 - 19
    Proximal Ulna: 20 - 21

W

Walther's Fracture: 210 - 211
Winquist Classification: 118 - 119

NOTES

ORDER FORM FOR HANDBOOKS

TITLE	PRICE x QUANTITY
Handbook of Common Orthopaedic Fractures, Second Edition (1992)	$ 14.00 x _____ = $ _____.__
Handbook of Commonly Prescribed Pediatric Drugs, Fourth Edition (1992)	$ 14.00 x _____ = $ _____.__
Handbook of Commonly Prescribed Drugs, Seventh Edition (Expected: Spring, 1992)	$ 14.00 x _____ = $ _____.__
Handbook of Commonly Prescribed Drugs, Sixth Edition (1991)	$ 13.50 x _____ = $ _____.__
Handbook of Commonly Prescribed Ocular Drugs (1991)	$ 13.00 x _____ = $ _____.__
Handbook on Pain Management, Third Edition (1991)	$ 13.50 x _____ = $ _____.__
Handbook of Over-the-Counter Preparations (1988)	$ 10.50 x _____ = $ _____.__
	SUB-TOTAL = $ _____.__
Shipping and Handling	= $ _3.00_
PA Residents: Add 6% Sales Tax	= $ _____.__
	TOTAL = $ _____.__

Send mail orders for Handbooks with checks or money orders to:

MEDICAL SURVEILLANCE INC.
P.O. Box 1629   West Chester, PA 19380

(PLEASE PRINT)

Name_____Degree_____

Organization_____

Street Address_____

City_____State_____Zip_____

Telephone Number_____

Signature_____

FOR FURTHER INFORMATION CALL COLLECT: 215 - 436-8881
FAX: 215 - 436-1803

ORDER FORM FOR COMPUTER DATABASES

TITLE	PRICE x QUANTITY
Pediatric DrugBase 1.0; Full Version (1992)*	$ 445.00 x ____ = $ _____.__
Pediatric DrugBase 1.0; Reduced Version (1992)*	$ 345.00 x ____ = $ _____.__
PA Residents: Add 6% Sales Tax	SUB-TOTAL = $ _____.__
	= $ _____.__
	TOTAL = $ _____.__

Check: Diskette Size ☐ 3.5" ☐ 5.25"

* *System Requirements:* To use Pediatric DrugBase 1.0, you must have an IBM or IBM compatible XT, AT or PS/2 computer (minimum 512 Kb of RAM memory). Software may be run with any version of DOS above 2.0; however, DOS 3.0 or higher is recommended. A hard drive is recommended for the fastest performance of the software. However, a hard drive is not required.

The price for either version includes: Program diskette(s), installation instructions, user manual, and a copy of the "Handbook of Commonly Prescribed Pediatric Drugs, Fourth Edition" (1992). Annual Pediatric DrugBase updates will be offered at a reduced price of $ 125.00 per year to buyers for two (2) consecutive years after the purchase of the program.

Send mail orders for Computer DataBases with checks or money orders to:

MEDICAL SURVEILLANCE INC.
P.O. Box 1629   West Chester, PA 19380

(PLEASE PRINT)

Name_____Degree_____

Organization_____

Street Address_____

City_____State_____Zip_____

Telephone Number_____

Signature_____

FOR FURTHER INFORMATION CALL COLLECT: 215 - 436-8881
FAX: 215 - 436-1803